The Musculoskeletal System in Children With Cerebral Palsy:
A Philosophical Approach to Management

Clinics in Developmental Medicine

The Musculoskeletal System in Children With Cerebral Palsy: A Philosophical Approach to Management

Martin Gough

Consultant Paediatric Orthopaedic Surgeon, Evelina London Children's Hospital,
Guy's and St Thomas' NHS Foundation Trust, London, UK

Adam Shortland

Consultant Clinical Scientist, Evelina London Children's Hospital,
Guy's and St Thomas' NHS Foundation Trust, London, UK

2022

Mac Keith Press

© 2022 Mac Keith Press

Managing Director: Ann-Marie Halligan
Senior Publishing Manager: Sally Wilkinson
Publishing and Marketing Co-ordinator: Paul Grossman
Production Manager: Andy Booth

First published in this edition in 2022 by Mac Keith Press
2nd Floor, Rankin Building, 139–143 Bermondsey Street, London, SE1 3UW

British Library Cataloguing-in-Publication data
A catalogue record for this book is available from the British Library

Cover designer: Marten Sealby

Cover image: The cover image reflects some of the themes of the book: two amorphous figures are either constructing or deconstructing a pile of bricks against a background of leaves. The book looks at how we need to form models of complex reality, how these need to be flexible and to change, and why it is important to avoid replacing one certainty with another. We also liked the colours.

ISBN: 978-1-911612-53-7

Typeset by Riverside Publishing Solutions Ltd
Printed by Jellyfish Solutions Ltd

Contents

Foreword   ix

Preface   xi

Acknowledgements   xiii

1. **What We Think and Why We Think It: Our Clinical Model of Cerebral Palsy**   **1**

   The Sound of Silence   3

   How Do We Know What We Know?   5

   Imposing a Structure on Sensory Information: Defining Our Own Reality   6

   System 1, Heuristics, and Bias   8

   Is All Knowledge the Same?   9

   Knowledge Within the Clinical Society   11

   The Concept of 'Spasticity'   13

   Does it Matter if There are Differing Concepts of Spasticity?   15

   The Role of Cognitive Dissonance   17

   Clinical Evidence and the Scientific Process: Is This Not an
      Objective Process?   18

   Thomas Kuhn and the Role of the Paradigm   19

   Factors Influencing Paradigm Change in a Clinical Society   21

   Moving Towards a New Paradigm   23

   The Objective Body and the Lived-In Body   26

2. **A Made-Up Story About Data, Knowledge, and Clinical Judgement**   **28**

   The Randomised Controlled Trial   30

   Sample Sizes and Outcome Statistics in Randomised Controlled Trials   30

   Bias in Randomised Controlled Trials   37

   Short-Term Follow-Up and Long-Term Outcomes   39

Clinical Guidelines   40
Summary and Recommendations   44

3. **The Musculoskeletal System: Not Just a Structure but a Process**   46
What is a System?   46
Linear and Nonlinear Systems   47
Cellos and Muscles   48
The Orchestra as an Example of a System   49
Considering the Human Musculoskeletal System as a Process
   Rather Than a Structure   50
Entropy, Information, and the Cell   51
The Cell Membrane: The Difference Between Inside and Outside the Cell   56
Proteins: The Workhorses of the Cell   56
How are Proteins Formed in the Cell?   57
Being a Cell Takes Energy   59
The Mitochondrion: The Cell's Power Station   59
Cellular Energy Balance   61
Systemic Energy Balance   62
A Cell is a Process as Well as a Structure   63
The Skeleton: More Than Just a Framework   63
Skeletal Muscle: The Prime Mover   65
The Myocyte: The Basic Biological Unit of Skeletal Muscle   65
The Components of Muscle Contraction   66
The Molecular Basis of Muscle Contraction   67
Muscle Architecture and Muscle Function   68
'Slow' and 'Fast' Muscles   70
Skeletal Muscle is Dynamic and Responsive   70
Muscle Innervation   72
Control of Movement: The Nervous System   72
The Neuron: The Basic Biological Unit of the Nervous System   72
The Basis of Neuronal Signalling: The Action Potential   73
Providing the Energy for Neuronal Signalling   74
The Concept of Upper and Lower Motor Neurons   75
The Central Nervous System Really is a System …   75
… And is Part of a Larger System Which Includes the Skeleton
   and Muscles   76
Interactions Within the Musculoskeletal System: Balancing Energy
   and Growth   77
Considering Musculoskeletal Growth as a Process   78

4. **Musculoskeletal System Development: Typical and Altered Trajectories**   **79**

Concepts in Cell Development: Epigenetics, State Space, and
   the Adaptive Possible   79

Considering Musculoskeletal Growth as a Trajectory   80

Entropy and Developmental Trajectories   83

This All Sounds a Bit Complicated …   84

Causal Loop Diagrams   85

Energy Costs of Growth   87

Musculoskeletal Development in the Embryo   88

Muscle Contraction Begins Early   89

The Role of the Corticospinal Tract   89

Movement and Motor Control After Birth   90

Skeletal Muscle Fibre Growth and Development   91

Factors Influencing Muscle Fibre Growth   92

Effect of Skeletal Muscle on Skeletal Development   93

Musculoskeletal Development in Children With Cerebral Palsy   95

Effect of Early Developmental Changes on Subsequent Musculoskeletal
   Growth and Development   96

Putting it All Together: Understanding and Exploring the
   Musculoskeletal System   99

Where Do We Go From Here?   100

5. **Evidence-Based Medicine and Cerebral Palsy**   **102**

Clinical Experience and Evidence-Based Medicine   103

The Problem with Randomised Controlled Trials in Cerebral Palsy   104

Summary of the Weaknesses of Evidence-Based Medicine When
   Applied to Cerebral Palsy   117

Building the Evidence for Treatment: Enhancing the Power of
   Observational Studies   117

Summary   124

6. **What Does All This Mean?**   **125**

Looking Again at How We View Clinical Knowledge   126

The Cynefin Framework and Knowledge Domains   127

Clinical Knowledge and the Cynefin Framework   130

Clinical Knowledge and Uncertainty   131

A Systems Approach to Clinical Knowledge   133

The Role of External Factors in System Development   135

Is This Helpful for Clinical Practice?   136

Critical Systems Heuristics   137
Sartre: Existence Comes Before Essence   141
Merleau-Ponty: We are Ensembles of Lived Meanings   142
The Clinical Relevance of the Lived-In Body   143
The Child With Severe Cognitive Impairment   144
The Lived-In Body as a Focus for Intervention   145
Putting Theory Into Practice   146
Does Life Really Need to be This Complicated?   152

Conclusion: Putting it Into Practice   154
References   156
Index   169

Foreword

Gough and Shortland shine a light on a number of areas of cerebral palsy that have been largely ignored hitherto. We do not fully understand the neuropathology for increased tone. Different definitions of spasticity have emerged – with different therapeutic implications. Are we sure what is primary and what is secondary pathology?

Working with a deficient theoretical base to say nothing of poor outcome data, it is not surprising that decisions to advise such interventions as physiotherapy, serial casting, botulinum toxin, and surgery vary widely among practitioners who nevertheless feel driven by therapeutic imperatives. We do not know how to take into account variability between children and their different circumstances.

Gough and Shortland confront these dilemmas head on. Given the muddle we are in, it is appropriate to start in Chapter 1 with how we know what we know, how that knowledge may be erroneous, how experience develops into concepts, how that knowledge can be shared, and the difficulty of application of knowledge to promote change in clinical practice.

They recognise that uncertainty is uncomfortable. They are in a fine tradition here. Ronnie Mac Keith embraced uncertainty directing his endeavours precisely to such areas.

In Chapter 2 they explore the limitations of the randomised controlled trial as currently practiced, interpreted, and applied in the context of cerebral palsy.

In Chapter 3 we are invited to consider the musculoskeletal system as a process rather than as a structure. Again we go back to basics with a discussion of entropy and how this relates to information flows within a network. This is followed by a comprehensive description of the structure and function of muscles and bones from the molecule upward, taking in energy generation and distribution along the way. They move to an exposition of innervation and the integration of muscle, bone, and adipose tissue as an endocrine system.

This is developed further in Chapter 4 with an emphasis on growth and development and how it may be altered in a child with cerebral palsy. Here we start with the stem cell, the gene regulatory network, and epigenetic influences. Development is envisaged as a variety of trajectories with a number of possible outcomes. With time, the number of possible options diminish – an effect which is discussed within the context of entropy which here reappears. This forms the basis for the introduction of causal loops, a number of examples of which illustrate the subsequent ideas. From the fertilised ovum we move through the migration of myoblasts to myotube development, myoneural innervations, the role of the corticospinal tract, muscle fibre growth and development, and the influence of muscles on the growing skeleton.

Cerebral palsy now emerges as the result of altered interaction within a complex adaptive system not solely the result of altered innervation but also receiving contributions from energy and nutritional depletion. The development of muscle pathology gives rise to secondary skeletal deformity.

How to move from the apparent complexity of this to apply it to the lived experience of the child is dealt with in Chapter 6.

Meanwhile Chapter 5 builds on Chapter 2. After further consideration of the limits of randomised controlled trials in the context of cerebral palsy, directed acyclic graphs are introduced as a tool for exposing the effects of confounding variables. It is suggested that combined with non-randomised longitudinal studies this would improve the quality of research as well as assist the transfer of knowledge from research to the clinic.

Before applying this, Chapter 6 first considers knowledge within the known/knowable/complex/chaotic Cynefin framework. Our experience and understanding of uncertainty can be incorporated into the framework of clinical system heuristics. This helps an understanding of how we make judgements about a system. This is illustrated by the application of this to a child with hip dysplasia. The concept of the 'lived in body' puts the child at the centre of any decision making.

A number of clinical vignettes first presented in Chapter 1 as illustrations of clinical confusion are represented here in the light of the ideas in the previous chapters. Goals are clarified, areas of uncertainty made explicit, and ways forward emerge.

You will not have read a book like this before. Intellectually fearless it is the product of wide reading and deep thought. Any student of biology cannot but be aware that what is known is but a small fraction of what is to be known. Confronted by the suffering of a child and family, Gough and Shortland open a space for us to pause and not rush to judgement. It is to be recommended to anyone involved in the management of children with cerebral palsy. There is also much food for thought here for those involved in decision making in a wider context.

Richard Robinson
Emeritus Professor of Paediatric Neurology,
Guy's, King's, and St Thomas' Hospitals, London, UK

Preface

A few years ago, we were very pleased to be invited to write a book on muscle function and growth in children with cerebral palsy, and on the associated implications for assessment and intervention. The objectives of the book were to review the current clinical model of musculoskeletal deformity in children with cerebral palsy, to discuss recent developments in our understanding of muscle and bone physiology, and to discuss alternative clinical models of assessment and intervention. We felt that the current clinical model was limited, and that the outcomes of intervention based on the model were limited, so these objectives seemed relatively straightforward until we started planning the book. We realised that to provide such a viewpoint for ourselves and for clinicians working within the current clinical model we needed to take a step outside the model to look at how we think about clinical models, to look at the evidence base for our clinical management, and to look at our model of the musculoskeletal system in children with cerebral palsy. As our understanding of these topics evolved, the book also evolved, and a new structure emerged which maintained the original objectives but placed them in a wider context. This is an enjoyable and exciting way to write a book but may not be the most efficient way to do so, and we are grateful for the forbearance and understanding of the editorial team at Mac Keith Press.

The resulting book has six chapters, followed by a short summary. Chapter 1 looks at how knowledge develops and becomes defined within an individual and within a society, with a particular focus on clinical knowledge. Chapter 2 takes these concepts and puts them in a practical context, that of the design and interpretation of a randomised clinical trial, generally considered as the gold standard for clinical evidence. Chapter 3 looks at the musculoskeletal system not as a structure but primarily as a complex adaptive system which involves interactions ranging from the cell to the community, and where movement and function are seen as emergent properties of these interactions. Chapter 4 looks at musculoskeletal system development, and helps us to consider how musculoskeletal growth may be altered in children with cerebral palsy. Chapter 5 looks at our current evidence base for clinical management and how our present approach does not encompass the challenge of individual variability. In Chapter 6, we consider clinical knowledge as a model we need to use to deal with a complex reality, discuss how such a model may benefit from a systems approach, and discuss how we may develop such a model within the context of the lived experience of the child with cerebral palsy. The summary discusses some further recommendations for the development of clinical models in this area.

On looking at the completed book, we realised that we had written the book we would have liked to have read before writing a better book, but realised also that even at Mac Keith Press forbearance and understanding may have limits. We hope that this book will act as a source of information and will provide new perspectives to facilitate discussion about our approach to the assessment and management of the musculoskeletal system in the child with cerebral palsy. We hope also that our book may encourage clinicians to consider how they think about the child with cerebral palsy, consider how they communicate these concepts within the clinical context, and consider how our thoughts and approach are shaped by the paradigm in which we act. In the words of the linguist Edward Sapir (1929: 207):

> Human beings do not live in the objective world alone, nor alone in the world of social activity as ordinarily understood, but are very much at the mercy of the particular language which has become the medium of expression for their society. It is quite an illusion to imagine that one adjusts to reality essentially without the use of language and that language is merely an incidental means of solving specific problems of communication or reflection. The fact of the matter is that the 'real world' is to a large extent unconsciously built upon the language habits of the group ... we see and hear and otherwise experience very largely as we do because the language habits of our community predispose certain choices of interpretation.

We appreciate that language acts as a form of verbal shorthand with which we discuss reality but may not always consider how our use of words may influence how and what we think and believe. In the child with cerebral palsy, for example, considering the terms child, muscle, bone, contracture, and function as being more like verbs than nouns can change our perspective on these concepts. We need to consider the child, their musculoskeletal system, and their environment as processes which change, develop, and interact. In the words of Ernest Fenollosa, art critic and historian (1920: 451):

> A true noun, an isolated thing, does not exist in nature. Things are only the terminal points, or rather the meeting points of actions, cross-sections cut through actions, snap-shots. Neither can a pure verb, an abstract motion, be possible in nature. The eye sees noun and verb as one: things in motion, motion in things.

Considering the musculoskeletal system in a child with cerebral palsy as a linked system of interactive processes and subsystems, extending from individual molecules to the child and their environment, may initially seem challenging but has the potential to open up a new approach to our understanding of growth and development of the musculoskeletal system in children with cerebral palsy, which can benefit the children and families we see. We hope that this book will contribute to this process.

Acknowledgements

To our wives and families, for their support and patience over the last few years while we wrote this book and for their confidence that we could finish it.

"It is ... particularly in periods of acknowledged crisis that scientists have turned to philosophical analysis as a device for unlocking the riddles of their field."

Kuhn 1970: 88

What We Think and Why We Think It

Our Clinical Model of Cerebral Palsy

Vignette 1: Eleanor

Eleanor is an experienced physiotherapist with a particular interest in the care of children with cerebral palsy. She is attending a clinical case discussion at an international academic meeting regarding possible surgical options for a child with cerebral palsy. Three leading surgeons discuss their preferred options; each surgeon appears confident and seems to view their approach as the most effective one. Eleanor notes that the surgical options advanced by the three surgeons are different. She wonders how each surgeon can be so confident about their approach and why they do not seem concerned that the other surgeons have a different approach. She wonders whether there is an objective 'best approach' or 'best practice', or whether a clinician's approach depends primarily on their experience and training. She wonders also whether the confidence of the surgeons is a response to an awareness of the apparent lack of an agreed and objective approach. She wonders perhaps most of all why the delegates at the meeting seem to accept the discussion and reported that they found it helpful.

Vignette 2: Sue

Sue is a postdoctoral researcher and is an expert on skeletal muscle function. She hopes to become involved in basic science research that will help the care of children with cerebral palsy and has attended a major clinical conference to gain a better understanding of the clinical issues and approach. She appreciates the enthusiasm and commitment of the delegates but is concerned that there appear to be intrinsic contradictions in the accepted treatment model, which essentially involves immobilising and denervating muscle with the aim of helping it to grow. She has noted also that a number of key clinical concepts discussed, such as the concept of spasticity, appear to be incompletely defined when used by the clinicians and appear to have a number of mutually incompatible definitions. She wonders how the clinical model developed and wonders whether the clinicians involved are aware of the inconsistencies within the model. She wonders also whether these issues may limit the development of further understanding of the underlying clinical problem.

Vignette 3: Mobin

Mobin is a physiotherapist looking after Colin, an 8-year-old boy with severe cerebral palsy. Mobin has worked very closely to help Colin to be as comfortable and functional as possible. On the advice of his senior physiotherapy colleagues, he has developed a postural management programme for Colin that involves the use of orthoses, a standing frame, and a sleep system with the aim of correcting Colin's existing lower limb deformities and preventing the development of further deformity. Colin has also had a number of episodes of serial casting and botulinum toxin injections. Mobin and Colin's parents are concerned that Colin appears to be getting stiffer and tighter and that he is finding the use of the orthoses and standing frame uncomfortable. Colin's parents have asked Mobin whether Colin needs to continue with his postural management as it is causing problems with his sleep and his mood. Mobin has previously assumed that this was the best approach but now has concerns that he may not be helping Colin and instead may be making things worse for Colin. He is concerned that if he continues with the present management he may cause Colin more pain, and is concerned that if he stops the present management he may be responsible for allowing Colin's deformities to proceed. He is worried and unsure how to proceed. He notes that his colleagues do not share his concerns and remain convinced of the efficacy of the treatment plan. Mobin wonders if he is missing something.

Vignette 4: Sara and Miguel

Sara and Miguel are the parents of Maria, a 4-year-old girl with bilateral cerebral palsy. They are concerned about her future independence and mobility. Maria currently takes some steps with the support of a posterior walker, and appears to be making progress in her mobility. Maria's physiotherapist has explained that Maria's walking ability is limited by something called spasticity, which her parents understand causes stiffness and discomfort in Maria's lower limbs and which prevents Maria's muscles from growing as they should. Maria's physiotherapist has discussed a treatment called selective dorsal rhizotomy, which she says can take spasticity away. Maria's parents have been in contact with a team in a hospital in another country who accept international referrals for selective dorsal rhizotomy. This team seem very positive about being able to help Maria to walk independently. Maria's paediatrician has known Maria and her parents since Maria was born and has been very supportive. He has advised caution regarding the potential benefit of selective dorsal rhizotomy for Maria, but when Maria's parents press him for information about Maria's future mobility, he does not seem to be able to give them the precise and definite prediction that they feel they need to be able to plan ahead. The treatment is very expensive, and it means putting Maria through surgery and extensive rehabilitation afterwards, but it seems to offer Maria the ability to walk independently. Maria's parents trust her paediatrician but he seems to be less positive in his approach than the team in the hospital and less definite about the outcome of surgery for Maria. The explanation from Maria's physiotherapist about the role and importance of spasticity makes sense to her parents and the positive approach of the surgical team is encouraging. Surely the team in the specialist hospital would not be as positive unless the treatment really worked as they said?

Vignette 5: Ana

Ana is a children's orthopaedic surgeon who has been monitoring the hip development of Peter, a 5-year-old boy with bilateral cerebral palsy. Peter has mild hip dysplasia, which does not appear to be progressing, and has significant medical comorbidities including problems with epilepsy, respiratory function, and gastro-oesophageal reflux. Ana's view has been that the risks of surgical intervention to his hips for Peter at present outweigh the likely benefits, and she has explained this to Peter's parents, Tom and Mary. They have been asking Ana for definite predictions about Peter's hips both in terms of his likelihood of progression of dysplasia and his risk of long-term hip pain. Ana has explained that this is difficult to precisely quantify. Tom and Mary have now contacted Ana to say that Tom will be having bilateral hip surgery done by another surgeon in a different hospital, following their request for a second surgical opinion. Tom and Mary have explained that the other surgeon seemed more confident and much more definite about what was likely to happen to Peter's hips without surgery, and showed them clear guidelines about the management of hip dysplasia in children with cerebral palsy. Ana is an experienced surgeon who has kept up to date with the published literature on hip dysplasia in children with cerebral palsy. She wonders why things do not seem as clear for her as they seemed to the other surgeon and wonders why she finds it difficult to give definite predictions of the natural history of hip dysplasia and the outcome of surgery for an individual child.

Vignette 6: Hans

Hans is a 12-year-old boy with bilateral cerebral palsy. He finds it increasingly difficult to walk with the support of his posterior walker; his legs become tired and uncomfortable, and his splints feel heavy. Hans has just started at secondary school and finds this difficult. The school is larger than his previous school and he has not made many friends yet. Hans feels self-conscious when he walks and thinks that people are looking at him. He finds his wheelchair is comfortable and finds it easier to get around in his wheelchair, but his parents and physiotherapist are keen for him to walk as much as he can.

Hans feels that he has had a lot done to his legs including physiotherapy, splinting, casting, botulinum toxin injections, and surgery. He has daily stretches, which are uncomfortable. His physiotherapist and his parents talk to him about 'spasticity' and 'core strength', and are discussing the use of a standing frame to stretch his legs and about the possibility of more surgery. Hans' friend Stella had surgery recently because she did not like the way her legs looked and because she thought that she might make friends more easily if her legs looked better and worked better. Stella has told Hans that her legs look straighter now, but she still has problems walking and still finds it hard to make friends. Hans does not think that he wants any more surgery. Hans knows that his parents and physiotherapist want to help him but wonders why everyone seems more interested in his legs than in him.

THE SOUND OF SILENCE

In August 1952, at a concert in Woodstock, New York, the pianist David Tudor gave the first performance of a new composition by John Cage, provisionally titled 'Four Pieces'. Placing the score on the piano, he started a stopwatch, closed the lid of the piano keyboard, and sat without moving for 33 seconds. He then opened and closed the keyboard lid again before sitting for 2 minutes 40 seconds. Following this, he closed the lid again before sitting for 1 minute 20 seconds. He then stood to mild applause from the remaining members of the audience before leaving the stage.

Following the concert, anger was expressed by the audience at what appeared to be a publicity stunt. When interviewed about the piece however, Cage (1968: 65) said:

> They missed the point. There's no such thing as silence. What they thought was silence, because they didn't know how to listen, was full of accidental sounds. You could hear the wind stirring outside during the first movement. During the second, raindrops began pattering the roof, and during the third the people themselves made all kinds of interesting sounds as they talked or walked out.

There have been a number of interpretations of the meaning or intent of the piece, which was subsequently known by its duration, 4′33″. These included an extended use of the silences normally found between sounds in music, a statement about the meaning of music itself, and a demonstration of the interest and beauty of what are considered ordinary sounds when we listen closely without prior preconceptions. Cage himself was not specific about an intended meaning of the piece but did give some ideas about what the piece meant for him. In an interview in 1989, 3 years before he died, he said 'No day goes by without my making use of that piece in my life and in my work. I listen to it every day … I don't sit down to do it; I turn my attention toward it. I realise that it's going on continuously' (Duckworth 1989: 21–22). In 1990 Cage wrote: '(S)ilence is … a change of mind, a turning around … silence was not the absence of sound' (Cage 1990).

Cage's biographer, Kay Larson, notes that there were three versions of the score for the piece: the final version, published in 1961, consisted of a sheet of paper with the following text:

I

TACET

II

TACET

III

TACET

'Tacet' is a Latin word meaning '(it) is silent', and is a musical term to mean that a particular instrument or voice should not sound. Prior to composing the piece, Cage had developed an interest in Zen Buddhism and had attended lectures in New York given by Dr Daisetz Suzuki. In these lectures Suzuki talked about how our consciousness imprints itself on everything we see and do. Larson (2012: 285) saw the score of 4′33″ as a proposition: 'It says, in notational shorthand: Stop for a moment and look around you and listen; stop and look; stop and listen.' If we see 4′33″ as a means of looking at underlying reality rather than viewing it through our preconceptions, this makes sense of Cage's comments above about his daily use of the piece, and his comments during the same interview with William Duckworth (1989):

DUCKWORTH: Well, the traditional understanding is that it opens you up to the sounds that exist around you and …

CAGE: … to the acceptance of anything, even when you have something as the basis. And that's how it's misunderstood.

DUCKWORTH: What's a better understanding of it?

CAGE: It opens you up to any possibility only when nothing is taken as the basis. But most people don't understand that, as far as I can tell.

The relevance of John Cage and 4′33″ to our understanding of the musculoskeletal system in the child with cerebral palsy, and to a philosophical analysis of our clinical approach, may not be obvious until we think about it. Like the audience in Woodstock with an expectation and preconception as to what constituted music, as clinicians we have preconceptions about the musculoskeletal system of the child with cerebral palsy that colour and perhaps limit our understanding, and that influence and constrain our approach to clinical management. A clinical 4′33″, if we could imagine such a process, would involve looking at the musculoskeletal system of the child with cerebral palsy without such preconceptions and without the need to apply a normative framework. Cage wrote that the composer 'must set about discovering a means to let sounds be themselves rather than vehicles for man-made theories' (1961: 10). He saw this as being a way to accept sounds for themselves: 'my silent piece … expresses the acceptance of whatever happens in that emptiness' (Kostelanetz 2003). As clinicians involved in the care of children with cerebral palsy, we could argue in a similar manner that the clinician must set about discovering a means to let children be themselves rather than vehicles for man-made theories, and work towards developing an acceptance and understanding of what is happening rather than impose our preconceptions.

Cage first mentioned the concept of a silent piece in 1948; he needed time for preparation and exploration before the piece was ready to be performed. In the same way, suggesting that we take a step back to look at the musculoskeletal system of the child with cerebral palsy without preconceptions involves time spent understanding what those preconceptions may be. This in turn involves understanding how clinical knowledge develops. These concepts may seem far removed from our everyday work as clinicians involved in the care of children with cerebral palsy, but as we have seen in the vignettes above, the basis of our clinical knowledge and how clinical knowledge develops and is shared are very relevant to our clinical practice.

In this chapter we will consider first how we view reality and how we think as individuals, and will then consider how knowledge is defined and shared within the clinical society. In Chapter 2, we will look more closely at sources of potential bias in clinical research. In Chapters 3 and 4, we will look at the musculoskeletal system as a complex adaptive system, and will consider the opportunities this offers to develop a clinical model of altered development in children with cerebral palsy. In Chapter 5, we will look again at how we view evidence and will discuss an approach to thinking about causation. In Chapter 6, we will draw these strands together to look again at a systems approach to clinical knowledge.

HOW DO WE KNOW WHAT WE KNOW?

What does it mean to know something? How do we agree on what we know? When does a concept become considered a fact? Where does clinical knowledge come from? How is it shared? What do we do if clinicians disagree? How does clinical knowledge change or develop?

Discussions regarding what constitutes reality and how we interpret it are likely to have been going on since we first developed language. In philosophy, this topic is termed 'metaphysics'. It is a challenging topic as there are a number of different concepts and definitions, and the terminology used can be somewhat bewildering to someone coming to it for the first time. Ontology (from the Greek word 'ontos', meaning 'being') asks the question 'what is reality?' Epistemology (from the Greek word 'episteme', meaning 'knowledge') asks how we know what reality is. In terms of ontology, the view that reality exists independently of any beliefs or perceptions is termed 'realism', while the view that reality is a product of our ideas or exists in the mind is termed 'idealism'. In terms of epistemology, rationalism is the view that knowledge may be derived from reasoning, independent of sensory information. Empiricism is the view that knowledge can only be obtained from sensory information.

Most clinicians are realists and empiricists, meaning that we consider that there is a reality from which we take in sensory data to provide a mental concept. The German philosopher Immanuel Kant (*A Critique of Pure Reason*, 1787) suggested that our perception of reality is determined by the way in which our mind handles sensory information (Tarnas 1996: 343):

> What man knows is a world permeated by his knowledge, and causality and the necessary laws of science are built into the framework of his cognition … In the act of human cognition, the mind does not conform to things; rather, things conform to the mind.

Kant made a distinction between a 'percept' and a 'concept' which is relevant to our discussion. In his terms, a percept is a sensory input, and a concept is our interpretation of that sensory input. If we look at a leaf, for example, we perceive reflected photons which have a wavelength of around 510nm and from this percept we form a concept of 'green', which we in turn associate with our concept of a 'leaf'. We will see later in the chapter how the distinction between a percept and a concept has a clinical relevance.

IMPOSING A STRUCTURE ON SENSORY INFORMATION: DEFINING OUR OWN REALITY

Imposing a structure on incoming sensory information and in this way limiting the amount of information that we take in is likely to reduce the amount of effort needed to analyse and interact with our environment. Our brains can take in much more information than we can actually handle in our consciousness. If we think of information in terms of bits, where each bit can be represented by a switch or signal that is on or off, Nørretranders estimated that our consciousness can handle up to 20 bits/second (Nørretranders 1991). He also, however, estimated that we perceive around 12 million bits/second (10 million bits from vision, 1 million bits from touch, and the remaining million bits from the other senses). This means that we are not able to consciously consider all the sensory information we receive. Having a means of condensing information into concepts or symbols allows us to think and respond to sensory inputs rather than drown in raw sensory data. As an example, when looking at the leaf mentioned above we receive input from a large number of photons distributed over a specific spatial distribution, but we 'see' a leaf rather than the signals from the individual photons. The ability to rapidly and selectively identify objects from a huge array of incoming sensory information, and the ability to rapidly form patterns and associations between these identified objects, are likely to have been very important in terms of survival and to have been refined through evolution. Being able to rapidly identify danger or assess a situation when there is limited data available may have been very important in determining survival for humans as a species; those who were able to rapidly identify a predator from a short glimpse with limited data, and take appropriate immediate action, are likely to have had a greater chance of survival than would have been the case if they had needed to wait until more data was available to form an interpretation of the situation.

Our ability to recognise patterns in the information presented to us and to rapidly construct theories or stories about what is happening from these patterns is discussed by Kahneman (2011). He suggested the concept of two different systems in the mind, which he termed System 1 and System 2. He emphasised that this was a concept to facilitate discussion, and was not intended to mean two structurally different systems. Kahneman suggested that System 1 is constantly active and reviews all sensory input on an ongoing basis to provide a continually updated picture of our current environment. System 1 allows us to recognise other people and almost immediately also recognise their mood, whether happy, angry, or sad. System 1 enables us to respond to sudden threats or dangers without needing to stop and consider them in detail, and can manage most simple tasks. System 1 can take in data, see patterns, and make associations to form a 'story', which can be presented to System 2. System 2 in comparison is used only when needed; it becomes involved when detailed concentration and focus on a specific cognitive challenge is needed as these tasks take more energy and are more effortful.

To get an idea of the difference between these systems, look at the following questions and try to come up with an answer for both before reading on:

$$1+1=?$$
$$127\times38=?$$

The first question is easy and does not require effort. It can be solved at a glance, even if we are doing something else. This question is answered by System 1. The second question is harder. To make an estimate of the answer it is necessary (for most of us!) to stop thinking about anything else, and focus specifically on the question. To mentally calculate the answer requires holding a number of items of information in memory during the successive stages of the calculation. This is tiring, and needs concentration; it would not be possible to answer this question when involved in another mental activity which needs concentration such as driving a car in heavy traffic.

Kahnemann suggested that in general we use System 2 only as needed and work predominantly with System 1. System 1 has the capacity to combine individual pieces of information to make a coherent picture: this picture is then presented to System 2. System 2 is not an independent or objective system; the focus of System 2 is directed by System

1, in the same way that our visual focus is directed by our peripheral vision. Kahneman suggests that the success of System 1, in terms of whether the information it presents to System 2 will be accepted, can be measured by the quality and coherence of the pattern or story System 1 has constructed from the data, and that the amount and quality of the data on which the story is based are largely irrelevant to System 2. He also suggests that the confidence that individuals have in their beliefs depends mostly on the quality of the story that these beliefs can tell. Data which appear to form or tell a story which is familiar and has been heard previously will lead to what Kahneman terms 'cognitive ease', while new and unfamiliar data may lead to 'cognitive strain'. Our judgement on whether the story we create from the data we receive is correct or not will be influenced by the associated cognitive ease or cognitive strain we perceive.

SYSTEM 1, HEURISTICS, AND BIAS

The data patterns and stories built up by System 1 are based on mental shortcuts termed 'heuristics'; these are generally very effective, particularly in social situations or in situations where there is danger, but may be less effective in some situations particularly where interpretation of more complex or numerical data is involved. In these cases they may result in a bias in data interpretation. Some of these biases are listed below (for more biases see Croskerry 2002; Elstein and Schwartz 2002); although these biases are relevant for all cognitive activities, they are discussed here in terms of clinical practice.

- **Confirmation bias:** the tendency for clinicians to look for information or data which is compatible with the opinion they currently hold rather than for information which will contradict their opinion.
- **Anchoring bias:** the tendency to fix on specific features of a presentation early in the diagnostic process and to base interpretation on this information: this can be a particular problem if linked with a confirmation bias as noted above.
- **Availability bias:** the tendency for things to be considered to be more frequent if they come readily to mind.
- **Representativeness bias:** judgement may depend on how well a clinical presentation matches the clinician's mental prototype for a particular diagnosis.
- **Commission bias:** tendency towards doing something rather than doing nothing (there is also an omission bias, which is a tendency towards inaction rather than action!)

Croskerry lists 27 different possible biases, including those listed above. This may be considered as discouraging and as a criticism of clinical practice but instead could be seen perhaps as an inevitable aspect of the way our brains can take in and integrate a huge amount of data, which may often be incomplete, and from this data formulate a working diagnosis and plan in a complex clinical situation (Croskerry 2002). The complexity of clinical problems and how we view and handle complex data will be discussed in more detail in Chapter 5.

A particular area in which we are prone to bias and to potential error is in the interpretation of numerical and statistical data. Kahneman discusses three different sequences of six births at a maternity hospital, where 'B' stands for boy and 'G' for girl; as the sex of the infant at each birth is not influenced by the sex of the previous birth these can all be considered as random sequences:

BBBGGG

GGGGGG

BBGBGB

Kahneman asks us if all sequences are equally likely; the answer is yes, but most people feel that the third sequence is most likely to represent a random sequence. We tend to dismiss the likelihood of a random event in the other sequences and instead look for an underlying pattern or cause. We are very good, as noted above, at seeing patterns in data and as a result can assume that random data is not random but is instead associated with an underlying cause. As an example, during the Second World War in 1944 around 2400 V-1 flying bombs landed on London. The impact site of each flying bomb was recorded. There was considerable concern following this as the data suggested clustering rather than a random distribution. Were the flying bombs being accurately guided to their destination or was this apparent clustering due to a random distribution? The data were reviewed by a statistician, DW Clarke, using a formula which is called the Poisson distribution (Clarke 1946). Clarke showed that despite the apparent clustering of the impacts of the flying bombs, the data did fit a Poisson distribution and the impact sites could be considered as random.

Kahneman discusses 'the law of small numbers' in his book and notes that small samples yield extreme results more often than large samples do. If a coin is tossed five times it may come up as heads rather than tails each time; if it is tossed 5000 times the ratio of heads to tails is likely to be closer to one. Our tendency to assume patterns in data which is randomly distributed and our lack of awareness of the greater variability in data from small samples as opposed to large samples can influence how we form hypotheses, and how we interpret data and will be discussed in more detail in later chapters.

IS ALL KNOWLEDGE THE SAME?

The data we take in is selected by our consciousness and then built into a model or construct which we consider as 'knowledge'. Knowledge is defined by the dictionary as facts, information, and skills acquired through experience or education. In the English language, the term knowledge is used in a number of different ways which are not always easy to define. Recorded discussion about knowledge goes back over 2000 years to Aristotle who suggested in the Nicomachean Ethics (350 BCE) that there were different types of knowledge (Aristotle 2004). He distinguished between 'sophia' (wisdom) and 'episteme' (knowledge), with the term sophia being used for knowledge about aspects of things which were unchanging, and the term episteme being used to describe knowledge about things which could be discovered or understood. He used the term techne for the knowledge or expertise involved in being able to carry out an activity effectively, particularly an activity involving a craft or skill. Building a house or carving a sculpture, for example, both involved a particular techne. Aristotle suggested also that through the experience of performing an act or skill we developed a mastery of the act or skill, which included not just the technical aspects of the skill but also judgement in executing the skill. He termed this ability 'phronesis'. Phronesis seems a valid concept when we consider the learned skill involved in, for example, performing a clinical examination or procedure but goes beyond this to include also the act of judging when and to what extent we perform a procedure.

A similar concept was suggested in the 1950s by a scientist called Michael Polanyi (Polanyi 1962). Polanyi developed the concept of codified (or explicit) and tacit (or implicit) knowledge. Polanyi wrote his book initially as a response to a theory advanced by Karl Popper, a philosopher of science. Popper had suggested (*The Logic of Scientific Discovery*, first published in 1934) that scientists worked objectively to disprove hypotheses, and had suggested that only theories which were open to being proved wrong, by data gained from experimentation or observation, could be considered as scientific (Popper 2002). Polanyi argued that scientists were not objective in the sense of being detached from data and the formulation of hypotheses but were instead driven to work towards a particular idea or theory by what he termed tacit knowledge. In Polanyi's view, tacit knowledge was knowledge which was held but could not be fully expressed, and which was built up through interaction and experience but which may not be possible to fully explain or codify. He gave the example of a radiologist learning to interpret a chest radiograph: from an initial perception of light and dark areas at the beginning of their training, the radiologist develops perceptual and conceptual skills to the point that they can look at a chest radiograph, see the lungs and associated structures, and identify a tumour. If asked in detail how they do this, they can start to explain but may struggle to provide the full details. In a similar manner, a surgeon in training will read the description of an operative exposure and the subsequent operative technique but the understanding of how this knowledge can be applied effectively will depend on tacit knowledge gained from experience of assisting a more experienced surgeon. Once the surgeon has completed their training, they will continue to develop their understanding of the indications for the procedure, the operative approach, and the operative procedure in a way that allows them to perform the surgery more effectively. It may be possible to discuss some of this improved understanding explicitly as 'codified knowledge', but some of the developments in their understanding may not be consciously apparent to the surgeon. This tacit knowledge is then passed on to a further surgical trainee through the shared experience of surgical procedures. Polanyi suggested that tacit knowledge extended beyond a particular skill; it also underlies our capacity to make effective judgements in complex situations. Our ability to explain or make explicit all the factors involved, for instance in making a clinical decision, may be difficult because of the implicit knowledge used in formulating the decision. This may be the case in particular when we are dealing with a complex clinical situation where available data is limited; this will be discussed in more detail in Chapter 5.

Tacit knowledge is useful but by definition we do not have a way of making it codified or explicit; because of this it may be difficult to measure or quantify. We recognise that an individual clinician is experienced but would struggle to find a quantifiable measure of this experience other than the duration of time that the clinician has been practicing. We can look for the evidence base underlying a clinician's practice, but Polanyi would argue that this evidence base can be seen as codified knowledge which is not an independent entity but is instead formulated and interpreted through the tacit knowledge of the clinician. This concept is implicit in the definition of evidence-based medicine (Sackett et al. 1996), which is seen as an interaction between the relevant scientific evidence, the judgement of the clinician, and the patient's values and preferences. The current hierarchy of evidence, with systematic reviews seen as best evidence followed by randomised controlled clinical trials, and with expert opinion as the lowest level of evidence, would appear to limit the role and effectiveness of tacit knowledge, but Polanyi argued that codified knowledge can only be interpreted in the context of tacit knowledge. In a randomised controlled trial, for example, the formulation of the hypothesis and the selection of variables, along with the confidence that we are controlling for all the variables except for the one being randomised, may be guided much more by our tacit knowledge than we realise. This will be discussed in more detail in the next chapter. This does not mean, however, that tacit knowledge is infallible; if considered as analogous to System 1 as outlined by Kahneman, it will be open to the same potential biases.

KNOWLEDGE WITHIN THE CLINICAL SOCIETY

So far, we have discussed how we take in and consider data as individuals. Knowledge, however, also has a social component; as we discussed in the preface, we share our under-standing and our concepts with others through the use of language. We are also able to share and agree on the conceptual models we use for the interpretation of reality. The power we have to share ideas and concepts through language is easily overlooked. If I ask you, as the reader, to imagine a pink elephant wearing blue shorts, juggling oranges, and riding a unicycle, an image will come to your mind, although you are unlikely to have seen such an image previously. The power of language means that we can share a concept (even if our individual images differ). In order for language to be able to achieve this, we need to share the accepted meanings of words and their usage. We learn these terms in childhood. We can tell a child that the leaf we discussed above is 'green' or that the sky is 'blue', and the child will accept these concepts as objective reality in the same way that they accept the concept of a leaf as objective reality. Words such as 'green', 'blue', and 'leaf', however, represent shared concepts or models which have been agreed linguistically and socially.

Is this discussion relevant to the clinical management of the musculoskeletal system in children with cerebral palsy? As clinicians, we consider ourselves to be working within an evidence-based framework and consider ourselves as members of a group within which clinical knowledge is shared and discussed objectively. We may not consider, however, that as a group we influence what we consider as knowledge and determine how this knowledge is defined and communicated in the language that we use. In the preface, we quoted the linguist Edward Sapir: the '"real world" is to a large extent unconsciously built upon the language habits of the group … we see and hear and otherwise experience very largely as we do because the language habits of our community predispose certain choices of interpretation' (Sapir 1929: 207). These choices of interpretation will influence both what we consider as knowledge and also what we consider as the evidence to support this knowledge.

The formulation and development of a shared concept of knowledge within a society was discussed by Berger and Luckmann (1966) who included medicine as an example of a society. If we consider clinicians to be a group of people sharing similar concepts, using shared and agreed terms and language, and with a shared aim, this concept of a clinical society would seem appropriate. The concept would include 'subuniverses' or groups within the overall society, as suggested by Berger and Luckmann, with shared identity and particular roles in the society, such as paediatric physiotherapists and paediatricians. The benefit of such a society would be the ability of the members of the society to agree on a model of cerebral palsy which could facilitate care and management of children with cerebral palsy, and which could be presented to clinicians entering the society in a way which allows them to apprehend concepts of the condition and its management. As with the different levels of complexity in which a leaf could be considered in the models discussed above, the clinical society can define and agree on different levels of complexity of the model as appropriate in different contexts. The understanding of cerebral palsy and its management by a medical student will reflect the overall concept of the condition within the society but will be a simpler and more easily accessible model than that which will be used by a paediatric neurologist. The reduction in complexity in the model used by the medical student as compared to the model used by the paediatric neurologist is likely to be associated with a loss of information, but this may be offset by the ability of the student to develop an overall concept of the condition that can be applied practically within a given context and which can subsequently be developed and extended.

How do we define these concepts within a society? Berger and Luckmann suggest that there are three stages involved in defining social knowledge. The first stage is externalisation, where there is an agreement within a group or society regarding an aspect of knowledge. In the second stage, this knowledge is then objectified, or considered to exist independently of the individuals who contributed to its formation. The last stage is internalisation, where this knowledge is passed on to clinicians entering the society and is accepted by them as objective knowledge. In a subsequent book (Berger 1967), Berger used the term 'nomos' to describe the knowledge, values, and ways of living within a society; the nomos is the result of human choice, but the society aims to persuade individuals that the nomos is objectively true and should be taken for granted. Berger suggested that 'the most important function of a society is nomization', and suggested that a nomos 'provides us with stability, predictability, (and) a frame of reference in which to live' (Berger 1967: 22–23) as opposed to the alternative 'anomy' which is associated with chaos. Berger was discussing a sociological theory of religion in his book, but the analogy could be equally applied to any society including the clinical society. The ability to present a shared model or concept of a complex reality within the clinical society, such as a model of the child with cerebral palsy, facilitates understanding and helps in the formulation of management approaches. Berger and Luckmann suggest, however, that this happens through the internalisation and subsequent objectification of these concepts within a society. In other words, concepts that are useful become viewed as objective facts and a useful model of reality can be perceived and interpreted instead as reality. It could be argued that this process forms the basis of what is termed evidence-based medicine.

One way of looking at the concepts held within a society and the means in which these concepts are shared would be to view the situation from the perspective of a clinician with an interest in the care of children with cerebral palsy who has just started working in this field. We can imagine that the clinician will have access to different sources of information about cerebral palsy. These sources will include what is seen as objective and evidence-based knowledge, and will also include knowledge derived from the experience and understanding of colleagues already working in the field. These sources would correspond to the codified and tacit types of knowledge discussed by Polanyi. Although we consider clinical practice to be primarily evidence-based, Berger and Luckmannn (1966: 22–23) suggested that:

> Theoretical knowledge is only a small and by no means the most important part of what passes for knowledge in a society … The primary knowledge about the institutional order is knowledge on the pretheoretical level. It is the sum total of 'what everybody knows' about a social world, an assemblage of maxims, morals, proverbial nuggets of wisdom, values and beliefs, myths and so forth.

This 'pretheoretical knowledge', when shared by colleagues, can be effective in facilitating a common understanding but may be difficult for the clinicians involved to formally express and may be difficult to objectively test. In this way, Berger and Luckmann's concept of 'pretheoretical knowledge' could be considered analogous to Polanyi's concept of tacit knowledge. Concepts may be passed on, from one clinician to another, which convey information that is not contained in the available and agreed theoretical (or codified) knowledge. Concepts which are not clear and which are not supported by the available evidence may, however, also be passed on and may be taken as objective information about the underlying problem, and used to inform clinical management.

The value of pretheoretical knowledge for a clinician entering a particular field may be the interaction and mutual support of the concepts involved. We think of 'facts' but we may not always consider that a remembered fact cannot exist in isolation but needs the context of related and supporting facts. Dennett illustrates this with a hypothetical story about a man who has had neurosurgery to alter specific synapses to create a memory of an older brother, in this case living in the state of Maine (Dennett 2013). When asked about his family, the individual involved will remember a brother in Maine but when he is unable to respond to questions about the name and age of his brother he will dismiss the memory of his brother as inaccurate. This awareness of interaction and of an overall context or frame of reference within which information or data can be viewed could be seen as the difference between 'information' and 'knowledge'. This frame of reference was described by Berger as the 'nomos' and was described by Kuhn (1970) as a 'paradigm'; this will be discussed in more detail later in the chapter.

THE CONCEPT OF 'SPASTICITY'

The discussion above can seem somewhat theoretical and unrelated to clinical practice: could clinicians really share a concept which is not clear and then use this concept to guide clinical practice? An example of such a concept would be the use of the term 'spasticity', which is widely used within the clinical society involved in the care of children with cerebral palsy. It can be argued that having such a term allows a concept to be shared and discussed between individual clinicians and with parents and children, and helps to guide clinical management. It can also be argued that a term or concept may not strictly need to have an explicit definition if the term is used by a group to refer to a specific concept known to the group. A concept which is tacit, for example, may be difficult to codify but may still be shared. Ludwig Wittgenstein, a philosopher with an interest in language, suggested that rather than trying to define the meaning of a word, we should look at how the word is used within a specific context (Wittgenstein 1953). He used the term 'language game' to express this concept, suggesting that although we may struggle to define a word we use, we know how it is used in practice, which implies an accepted and agreed understanding of the word or term. He used the term 'game' as an example, noting that the term was used to cover children's games, sports, word games and games such as chess. While we may have difficulty in providing a definition that covers all aspects of use of the term 'game', we have an understanding of how the term 'game' is used and in this way what the term means. Is this the case with the concept of spasticity?

The term 'spasticity', as discussed within the clinical society, appears to be used in different ways and with different meanings. One aspect of its use appears to refer to a physical sign noted on clinical examination, while another aspect of its use appears to refer to an underlying clinicopathological process in the child. These aspects are frequently combined: the concept of treatment of spasticity is discussed, in which intervention to alter the physical sign assumed to be related to, or to represent, spasticity is performed in order to positively influence the underlying condition which is also assumed to be related to spasticity. The alteration in the clinical sign may then be assumed to represent an alteration in the underlying clinical condition. Both aspects of the use of the term contain ambiguity and in view of the widespread use of the term 'spasticity' it may be useful to explore this ambiguity further.

We can look first at the clinical finding of spasticity, which is based on examination. A clinician entering this field and asking colleagues for information about the definition and clinical measurement of spasticity may hear at least two different possible views in that spasticity may be presented as a velocity-dependent resistance of a muscle to stretch, or as a persistent activation of muscles.

The definition of spasticity as a velocity-dependent resistance to stretch of a muscle is derived from the more complete definition suggested by Lance, who stated that (Lance 1980: 1303):

Spasticity is a motor disorder characterised by a velocity-dependent increase in tonic stretch reflexes ('muscle tone') with exaggerated tendon jerks, resulting from hyperexcitability of the stretch reflex, as one component of the upper motor neuron syndrome.

Lance subsequently noted that (Lance 1990: 606):

Spasticity does not include impaired voluntary movement and an abnormal posture. These are often features of upper motor neuron lesions, as are other symptoms such as flexor spasms, and may be associated with spasticity but do not define it.

More recently, spasticity has been defined by Pandyan (Pandyan et al. 2005: 2–6):

Spasticity may be redefined as disordered sensori-motor control, resulting from an upper motor neuron lesion, presenting as intermittent or sustained involuntary activation of muscles.

The reader will note that the definition suggested by Lance specifically excludes impaired voluntary movement within the definition of spasticity while the definition suggested by Pandyan specifically includes impaired motor control. It is not clear whether one definition or the other is more widely accepted within the clinical society, whether a combination of both definitions is used, or whether other alternative concepts are used. Malhotra et al. reviewed 250 publications on spasticity and noted that 31% of the publications used the Lance definition of spasticity, 35% used a definition based on muscle tone, 3% used an alternative definition, and 31% of the publications related to spasticity did not define what was meant by spasticity (Malhotra et al. 2009).

The clinical method of assessment of spasticity is also variable; Scholtes et al. reviewed 119 published studies on spasticity and noted that 13 different assessment methods were used (Scholtes et al. 2006). The main types of assessment used were described as 'Ashworth-like', where an assessment of joint stiffness was used, and 'Tardieu-like', where an assessment of the effect of movement at different velocities on joint stiffness was performed. They concluded that most instruments do not comply with the concept of spasticity, that standardisation of the assessment method is often lacking, and that the scoring systems of most methods of assessment are ambiguous. This was noted also by Malhotra et al., who concluded that measures of spasticity often did not correspond to the definition of spasticity used, by which they meant that a measure of stiffness such as the Ashworth scale was used when spasticity was defined according to the Lance definition by the clinician performing the clinical examination, or a measure of the effect of velocity on stiffness was used where the definition was related to a perceived alteration in muscle tone. These can seem like minor points, but they indicate a fundamental ambiguity and confusion in our definition of spasticity as a clinical sign. Both the Lance and Pandyan definitions of spasticity imply an overlap between the clinical sign and the underlying clinical process, with the resulting implication that intervention to alter the clinical sign may alter the underlying process. Both definitions are presented as definitive descriptions of an underlying reality rather than as models of a complex process.

DOES IT MATTER IF THERE ARE DIFFERING CONCEPTS OF SPASTICITY?

Cerebral palsy is a complex condition and having useful and effective models of the underlying process which can guide management is important. When there is a lack of consistency or agreement within our approach, with acceptance of at least two contradictory models of spasticity with each seen as objectively factual, this cannot be good for clinicians working in the field or for clinicians entering the field and looking for guidance. It is likely that with experience, clinicians develop an individual model and definition which they find effective, but while this may be effective on an individual basis the current use of the term spasticity is reminiscent of the passage from Lewis Carroll's *Through the Looking-Glass*:

> 'When I use a word,' Humpty Dumpty said, in rather a scornful tone, 'it means just what I choose it to mean – neither more nor less.'

> 'The question is,' said Alice, 'whether you can make words mean so many different things.'

Part of the difficulty in defining and interpreting spasticity may be related to a confusion between models of reality and reality itself. We looked earlier at Kant's use of the terms 'percept' and 'concept'; Kant suggested that a percept is a sensory input, and a concept is our interpretation of that sensory input. The concept of spasticity is a model we use to manage a complex clinical problem, but it is essentially only a model; 'spasticity' as such is a mental construct we use. It could be said that spasticity as we define it exists in our minds rather than in the child being examined. This may not in itself be a problem as long as we are aware of how we are thinking, but can be a problem if we assume that our model of reality and reality itself are the same, and if we uncritically project our concept onto the child being examined. It may also be that as the term 'spasticity' is a noun we assume that it represents something that exists which can be experienced and quantified, rather than a mental representation. This is not an argument against the use of a clinical concept or model but instead a suggestion that caution be used in any interpretation of a clinical situation. As an example, a different degree of resistance of a muscle to stretch at different velocities of stretch may be interpreted as spasticity but may also simply reflect the altered compliance of muscle in children with cerebral palsy in comparison to the muscles of typically developing children. Willerslev-Olsen et al., for example, noted an alteration in the passive properties of muscle in children with cerebral palsy who were less than 3 years old; this was not related to an alteration in reflex response to stretch or active muscle contraction, and instead appeared to be due to an alteration in the intrinsic properties of muscle in these children (Willerslev-Olsen et al. 2013). Assessment of these muscles using our current approach would have led to a finding of 'spasticity' and to intervention to reduce this assumed spasticity with the goal of improving muscle growth and hence function. The interventions performed to reduce spasticity include immobilisation or denervation of a growing muscle, and a reduction in sensory input from the muscle through section of sensory nerve roots in the spinal cord. The model in use which guides these interventions involves the concept that passive stretch is important for muscle growth, and that spasticity limits the capacity of a muscle to respond to passive stretch and in this way limits or prevents muscle growth. Muscle growth and the development of musculoskeletal deformity in children with cerebral palsy will be discussed in Chapter 3, but it seems appropriate to say at this point that our current understanding of muscle growth does not suggest that passive stretch, as distinct from stretch imposed during active muscle contraction, is important in muscle growth. It appears instead that the main factors influencing early muscle growth and muscle fibre type differentiation are the development of an appropriate pattern of muscle innervation, adequate availability of muscle stem cells, and an environment where cellular energy is sufficient. It thus appears that our present model for the management of musculoskeletal deformity involves the treatment of a mental concept which does not have an agreed definition, is difficult to quantify clinically, which does not appear to be a cause of muscle deformity, and which is more likely to be an epiphenomenon than an independent entity.

The reader may ask that if this is the case, why is there still such an emphasis on the assessment and management of spasticity in children with cerebral palsy within the clinical society? There are likely to be a number of reasons. The main reason, as noted above, may be that within the clinical society the concept of spasticity has become viewed as objective or factual knowledge in the manner outlined by Berger and Luckman. It may also be related to what Kahneman describes as 'cognitive ease'. Kahneman suggested that the measure of success we employ for our System 1 is the coherence of the story it manages to create for System 2 and the frequency with which we are presented with this story, and suggests that the amount and quality of the data on which the story presented to System 2 are based are largely irrelevant. The concept that muscle growth is related to passive muscle stretch, and that spasticity is something that limits the ability of the muscle to be stretched and hence to grow, may be seen as an appealing model which offers both a hypothesis regarding the mechanism underlying the development of deformity and a potential target for intervention. It allows a complex clinical problem to be managed in a way that can be shared and agreed by the clinicians involved. A critical reader coming to this topic could ask, however, why the term and concept of spasticity continue to be used, and continue to define our treatment model, given the inherent ambiguity discussed above. This may in part be explained by the concept of cognitive dissonance.

THE ROLE OF COGNITIVE DISSONANCE

The term 'cognitive dissonance' was introduced by Leon Festinger who suggested that as human beings we strive for internal psychological consistency in order to function optimally in the world. Cognitive dissonance occurs when we hold contradictory views or are exposed to new information which challenges our views. This dissonance is resolved by either changing our internal view or by modifying our understanding of the new or contradictory information so that it fits our existing view.

The most well-known example of cognitive dissonance described by Festinger was that of a group called the Seekers, led by Dorothy Martin, whose members were convinced that the Earth would be destroyed on a specific time and date, 00:00 on 21st December 1954, by a great flood (Festinger, Riecken, and Schachter 2017). They also believed that the members of the group would be rescued before midnight by a flying saucer, which would come from a planet called Clarion, the inhabitants of which had sent a message to this effect to Martin via automatic writing. The group members left their jobs and spouses, and gave away their possessions before meeting in Martin's house on the evening of 20th December. Festinger and his colleagues had infiltrated the group and reported events. After midnight there was increasing concern within the group until 04:45 when Martin stated that she had received another message via automatic writing to say that the group, by sitting all night, had spread so much light that the God of Earth had saved the world from destruction. Rather than a loss of conviction in their belief following the non-appearance of the flying saucer and the flood, the group members reported an increase in the strength of their convictions, and later that day the group contacted the newspapers to ask for interviews to spread the message and to spread their belief.

Festinger listed five conditions needed for an increase in belief after a failure of the belief or a disconfirmation of the belief:

- The belief must be held with deep conviction and be relevant to what the believer does.
- The person holding the belief must have committed to it, in other words taken some action based on the belief.

- The belief must be sufficiently specific that it can be refuted by events.
- This disconfirmatory evidence must occur and must be recognised by the individual holding the belief.
- The individual believer must have social support.

The example of the Seekers is somewhat extreme but illustrates the concept of cognitive dissonance well; at a less extreme level, the same mechanism may act within a clinical society. It may be difficult, for example, for an external objective reviewer (if such a being does exist!) to understand how muscle denervation by botulinum toxin or immobilisation of muscle by orthoses can help muscle growth, how reduction of sensory input from the lower limbs by selective dorsal rhizotomy may improve motor function, or how altering the alignment of the lower limbs by surgical intervention may significantly improve function in the presence of persisting problems with motor control and muscle strength. It may also be difficult for an observer to understand why some clinical approaches continue to be used without convincing evidence that they are effective in improving function. Some of the factors which underlie this approach may be the desire on the part of the clinicians to do something for the child with cerebral palsy, and to consider cerebral palsy (or 'spasticity') as a problem which can be successfully treated. This approach may allow the avoidance of uncertainty and avoidance of the underlying worry that we do not fully understand the problem and do not have an effective answer for these children. It is possible in this context that large academic meetings within the clinical society function primarily as a way of reinforcing conviction and belief in the model held by the society, and viewed by the clinical society as objective reality, by presenting a 'nomos' for the society. This will be effective in providing a unified approach which can help avoid uncertainty but may limit progress in understanding of the underlying condition within the clinical society. Senior clinicians who have devoted considerable time and effort to developing their practice, and who would be seen as leaders within the clinical society, may be particularly at risk of cognitive dissonance on the basis of Festinger's conditions as listed above; this may in turn explain their favourable interpretation of adverse intervention outcomes and may limit or prevent informed development of clinical practice within the clinical society as a result.

CLINICAL EVIDENCE AND THE SCIENTIFIC PROCESS: IS THIS NOT AN OBJECTIVE PROCESS?

It could be argued in response to the discussion above that the concepts held by the clinical society are informed by the evidence gathered through the scientific process, and are therefore in this way evidence based. The scientific method is extremely powerful; a hypothesis is formulated and is empirically tested to see if the findings match the model and in this way support or contradict the hypothesis which has been advanced. Discussion of the scientific method, however, often omits discussion of the observer who formulates the hypothesis, who chooses what to study and how to study it, and who interprets the data. This concern was discussed by Polanyi, as noted earlier, and other philosophers have advanced similar ideas. The Duheim-Quine thesis or Duheim-Quine problem (so called after Pierre Duheim and Willard Van Orman Quine, both of whom seem to have stated different theses) states that it is not possible to test a hypothesis in isolation, as testing a hypothesis involves background assumptions that other associated hypotheses involved are correct. A hypothesis is tested within an overall intellectual framework or system which is shared by the scientists working in that area. In a way that is similar to how knowledge can be constructed within a society as suggested above by Berger and Luckmann, the shared concepts and understanding of the scientific society (both codified and tacit) influence the formulation of hypotheses and the interpretation of data within the scientific society (Berger and Luckmann 1966). This had been suggested previously by Ludwik Fleck (1979), who used the terms 'denkkolectiv' (thought collective) and 'denkstil' (thought style) to suggest such a shared view, and who argued that a pure and direct observation cannot exist and that the observer is always influenced by the epoch and environment to which he belongs. Fleck also suggested that a scientific 'truth' was a relative value which depended on the thought collective within which it had arisen. He suggested also that thought collectives could become resistant to change or to displacement by opposing thought collectives, with the prevailing thought collective becoming a 'thought constraint' which then resists any progress or change.

This concept was echoed more recently by Jacques Derrida (Derrida 1977: 136) who stated:

> What is called 'objectivity', scientific for instance ... imposes itself only within a context which is extremely vast, old, firmly established, or rooted in a network of conventions ... and yet which still remains a context.

THOMAS KUHN AND THE ROLE OF THE PARADIGM

The work of Fleck and of Polanyi influenced the more well-known work of Thomas Kuhn who wrote *The Structure of Scientific Revolutions* in 1962 (Kuhn 1970). Kuhn argued that the common concept of scientific development as being a continuous linear process, with individual scientists adding information to build up our knowledge in a progressive fashion, almost like individual bricks being added to a wall, did not fit what has happened historically where existing prior concepts became superseded by new concepts. Kuhn used the term 'paradigm' to describe a shared scientific theory or model which is able to guide subsequent research. He stated that 'To be accepted as a paradigm, a theory must seem better than its competitors, but it need not, and in fact never does, explain all the facts with which it can be confronted' (Kuhn 1970: 17–18). The paradigm in Kuhn's view essentially defines and limits what form the associated research will take and what topics will be studied.

Although the concept of a paradigm can be seen as restrictive, Kuhn (1970: 24) suggested that through the associated focus of scientific effort on a specific area, 'the paradigm forces scientists to investigate some part of nature in a detail and depth which would otherwise be unimaginable'. He suggested that the study of these paradigms prepares the student for membership in a specific scientific community where the student will join scientists who share the same fundamental concepts, based on the same paradigms, and suggested that this agreement and the apparent consensus produced are prerequisites for what he called 'normal science'. By normal science, Kuhn meant the work done by scientists to further investigate and extend the existing paradigm. He suggested that experimental data which is obtained by scientists working within a paradigm will be interpreted in a way which is consistent with the paradigm, even if the data does not support the paradigm. Data may, however, accumulate which suggests that the existing paradigm may not be the most appropriate model, in which case there will be a period of uncertainty or model crisis. Kuhn noted that with increasing research within a paradigm, the limitations of the paradigm may become more apparent but suggested that initially efforts to resolve any perceived conflict between the data and the paradigm will be made while closely following the paradigm. If these efforts are successful, 'normal science' will resume. If not, he suggested that adjustments of the paradigm may occur; these may increase in number and may provide divergent interpretations of the original paradigm. These divergent interpretations may gain a basis of support from different parts of the scientific group, but there then may be confusion about the overall paradigm. He described this as a period of crisis within a paradigm which is followed by what he termed 'revolutionary science', where alternatives to an existing paradigm are explored. In some cases, this may lead to the adoption of a new paradigm. He termed this process a 'paradigm shift' and described the process as 'a reconstruction of the field from new fundamentals … when the transition is complete, the profession will have changed its view of the field, its methods, and its goals' (Kuhn 1970: 85).

Kuhn suggested that developments in science such as the move from the Ptolemaic view of the universe, where the Earth was considered to be at the centre of the universe and the sun and stars were considered to revolve around it, to the Copernican view of the universe where the Earth was considered to revolve around the sun, was an example of a paradigm shift. The move from the classical Newtonian model of reality, which involved an invariant and constant time and space, to Einstein's theory of relativity was seen by Kuhn as another example of a paradigm shift. In each case, the competing theories are different in terms of the model used and in terms of how the data is interpreted to the extent that they can be viewed as different world views. A scientist can work within only one paradigm and will not be able to compare two paradigms objectively. Kuhn termed this 'incommensurability'. One way of understanding the concept of incommensurability may be to consider a paradigm as similar to Berger's concept of the 'nomos' as discussed earlier. If the society is effective the nomos will be seen as objectively true and will be taken for granted, meaning that there can only be one nomos within a society at a given time.

A new paradigm may be accepted if it solves a recognised problem and if it is likely to preserve a great deal of the achievements of the existing paradigm. Kuhn noted that in its initial stages, a new paradigm will be less detailed than the existing paradigm but will have significant promise for future problem solving. Kuhn (1970: 155) suggested that the reason some scientists became interested in a new paradigm shift was not defined fully by logical analysis but instead was influenced by 'arguments, rarely made entirely explicit, that appeal to the individual's sense of the appropriate or the aesthetic – the new theory is said to be "neater", "more suitable", or "simpler" than the old'. This idea drew criticism from scientists and from philosophers of science such as Karl Popper when the book was published as it suggested that there may be irrationality at the centre of the scientific method, but from the earlier discussion of Polanyi's work the adoption of a new paradigm could instead be seen as an interaction between tacit and codified knowledge. It could also be viewed as a shift within the scientific group or society from one overall belief system to another in which the same data is viewed and interpreted in a different manner.

In the context of the management of the musculoskeletal system in children with cerebral palsy, the concept of spasticity and its role in the development of musculoskeletal deformity, together with the concepts relating to the assessment and treatment of spasticity, could be seen as our current clinical paradigm. Viewed from within, possibly with the benefit of both cognitive ease related to the familiarity of the model and cognitive dissonance in relation to ambiguities within the model and the lack of positive outcomes from intervention to what is viewed as spasticity, the paradigm provides a framework within which clinical management is guided and research is designed and interpreted. If we take a step back, however, the current paradigm would appear to be entering a state of crisis with divergent articulations of the underlying concept, a lack of agreement within the clinical society regarding interpretation or definition of the concept, and a lack of progress as regards the outcomes of clinical intervention.

FACTORS INFLUENCING PARADIGM CHANGE IN A CLINICAL SOCIETY

The potential crisis of the existing paradigm may take some time to influence current clinical practice as the clinical society is not primarily a scientific society. This is not to suggest that the clinical society is not scientific but instead that, as suggested by Berger and Luckmann, the knowledge defined and shared by the clinical society will include theoretical and pretheoretical knowledge, in other words both scientific sources of evidence and 'what everybody knows'. This is in a sense comparable to the tacit and codified elements of knowledge as described by Polanyi. Within a clinical society there may be limited crossover or translation of codified knowledge to knowledge which is tacit or implicit. The tacit knowledge of a clinician, obtained from clinical experience and passed on to colleagues and trainees, is valuable in terms of helping the clinician to work with huge amounts of raw data in a complex situation, and can effectively inform the clinical practice of the clinician involved and subsequently of their trainees. The difficulty is that this tacit knowledge is difficult to quantify objectively and as it is difficult to codify it may be difficult to share explicitly. There may also be variation or differences in the tacit knowledge of different clinicians, with the tacit knowledge of an individual clinician being influenced by their training and experience. It is possible for tacit knowledge to be shared within an institution but to differ from the tacit knowledge shared within another institution. The tacit knowledge will influence the interpretation of available evidence or codified knowledge so that an individual clinician may interpret a published research paper, for example, from the viewpoint of his tacit knowledge. Clinical decision-making may also, as will be discussed in later chapters, be influenced by limitations of the available evidence in terms of the methodology used in obtaining and analysing experimental data.

Interpretation of published research will also be influenced by cognitive dissonance as discussed earlier. A senior clinician who has devoted their career to the development of a particular approach which has guided their clinical decision-making, and which has involved the use of treatment such as botulinum toxin injections which would not be supported by a different paradigm, may have an unconscious bias against change. This may result in a situation where two clinicians may express contrasting views regarding clinical management, with each view being supported by a combination of individual experience and individual interpretation of available published evidence. This can lead to variation in data interpretation and subsequent treatment recommendations made by clinicians. Skaggs et al. reported on the interpretation of gait analysis data from seven children by 12 experienced physicians from six institutions (Skaggs et al. 2000). They concluded that the identification of problems from physicians from the same institution tended to be more similar than between institutions, and noted that following interpretation of the same data one child would be five times more likely to have bone surgery recommended at one institution in the study than would be the case at another institution. This is not a situation exclusive to the management of children with cerebral palsy. Lindsey and Newhouse (Lindsey and Newhouse 1989) prepared a report for the US Department of Health and Human Services on the Second Surgical Opinion Program. This programme enabled a patient for whom surgery had been recommended by one surgeon to have a second opinion from another surgeon. Lindsey and Newhouse noted that high non-confirmation rates (where the second opinion differs from the first) 'signify a different opinion, but not necessarily a more valid one'. The same process was reviewed by Rutkow et al. (Rutkow, Gittelsohn, and Zuidema 1979). They concluded that 'surgical decision making is a semi-exact scientific process, and it is unreasonable to expect exact answers to clinical problems'. They noted that the study did not examine the interpersonal factors involved in the relationship between the surgeon and the patients which may also have influenced the surgical decision made.

These studies discuss surgical decision-making but similar findings have been reported in the case of medical or non-operative decision-making. As we have discussed, the difference in opinion is likely to be related to differing interpretations of the available evidence and to differences in clinical experience and in the subsequent internalisation of this experience by individual clinicians. The process may be influenced also by an awareness of the underlying uncertainty of clinical practice and the expectation on the part of the family and society that a clinician should be knowledgeable and should make the correct clinical decision in a given situation. In such a situation, excessive confidence in clinical decision-making may mask underlying concern about the validity of the clinical model and an associated element of uncertainty. If this occurs, any apparent challenge of the clinician's decision by the family, or by other clinicians, may result in defensiveness on the part of the clinician. A more pragmatic approach for the clinician would be to discuss the uncertainty inherent in clinical decision-making with the family. There is limited evidence available, however, as to how this would be perceived by parents and children, and there may be a reluctance among clinicians to take this approach. These concepts are discussed in more detail in Chapter 5.

A review of our current position as a clinical society involved in the management and care of children with cerebral palsy suggests that although we have an agreed paradigm within the society regarding our understanding of the mechanism of musculoskeletal deformity and the appropriate protocols for intervention, this paradigm is in crisis with a number of different and competing interpretations of the core concept of spasticity and with a lack of evidence to support some of the current intervention options we use. The concepts we share about the underlying clinical problems, such as spasticity, are necessarily simplified cognitive models which we use to view or consider children with a complex clinical problem. These models facilitate our understanding and help us to formulate a therapeutic approach but are still just models. This approach can lead to a focus on the assessment of impairments such as spasticity and on intervention to reduce these impairments, and can lead to a reduced focus on how our models relate to the functional status and the quality of life of the children we see. This is not to say that the model or paradigm that we use does not have some effectiveness and utility in informing clinical management; if it did not have some utility and did not possess an inherent and persuasive coherence, it is unlikely to have been adopted in the first place. Because of this, bringing about a change in the nomos or paradigm within a clinical society may not be easy. The current paradigm is familiar and may be interpreted within the society as objective or externalised knowledge which has informed clinical practice and is widely shared. The introduction of a different view, and the suggestion that the core concepts of the clinical society are cognitive concepts rather than objective facts, are likely to cause cognitive dissonance for some members of the clinical society. The factors listed by Festinger as being responsible for an increase in belief after a disconfirmation of this belief would appear to be equally applicable in this situation. There may be a concern that relinquishing our current model or nomos and accepting uncertainty may, as Berger has suggested, give rise to 'anomy' or chaos. There may be a perception that having a model which works to some extent is better than not having a model at all. The challenge will be to bring the clinical society and the families forward together while maintaining the close relationship which exists. There are a number of ways in which this could occur, and these are discussed below. They are presented in a particular order for the purpose of discussion but could happen in an alternate order or could happen simultaneously. The approaches discussed are covered in more detail in the next chapters but are summarised here for convenience.

MOVING TOWARDS A NEW PARADIGM

A first step may be for us to formally recognise and accept the uncertainty and lack of knowledge in our current understanding of musculoskeletal function and growth in children with cerebral palsy. This does not mean that we say that we do not know anything, but instead that we appreciate the limitations of our present knowledge and communicate these limits with the children and parents we see. As an example, if we see a child with mild hip dysplasia we can predict whether this may progress on a population basis, but we do not have the understanding to make an accurate individual prediction. This concept will be discussed in more detail in Chapter 5. In a similar manner, if asked whether and when musculoskeletal deformities will recur following surgery, we do not have the understanding or capacity to make an accurate prediction in an individual but instead rely on an estimate based on experience, essentially using our tacit knowledge. Acceptance of the limitations of our understanding does not mean that we cannot plan an intervention and discuss this with the child and family; instead, by discussing and admitting our limitations in knowledge we invite discussion and participation on the part of the child and family so that the treatment plan becomes a joint agreement with a greater awareness of the knowledge context within which the agreement has been made. As we will discuss in Chapter 6, certainty is an extreme position; it is possible to be 99% certain but by definition to still be uncertain.

It is possible that some parents (and some clinicians) may not be happy with the suggestion that clinical practice is not as evidence-based as they would wish, and that there are things that as clinicians we do not fully know or cannot accurately predict. A discussion based on the assumption that we do have all the information would not, however comforting it may be for the parents and clinician, be in the best interests of the child. As clinicians we are used to dealing with complex problems and with uncertainty; an explicit acceptance of this by the clinical society is likely to be favourably received by most clinicians. Maurice Merleau-Ponty, a French philosopher, gave a lecture in 1953 (In Praise of Philosophy) where he stated that 'the philosopher is marked by the distinguishing trait that he possesses inseparably the taste for evidence and the feeling for ambiguity' (Merleau-Ponty 1988). He envisioned a constant movement between the two, 'which leads back without ceasing from knowledge to ignorance, from ignorance to knowledge'. The same concept was expressed also by an American poet, EE Cummings: 'all ignorance toboggans into know, and trudges up to ignorance again' (Cummings 1991). As clinicians we share this trait and this feeling; when considering what we know, we become more aware of what we do not know, and when considering what we do not know, we become more aware of what we do know. In this way knowledge can be seen not as a fixed entity but instead as a changing and developing process; this concept will be explored further in Chapter 6.

The next step in moving towards a new paradigm would be to look at the concepts we use when we consider and discuss the musculoskeletal system in children with cerebral palsy, and how these concepts are expressed through language. It may be unrealistic to expect that a consensus will rapidly develop within the clinical society regarding a concept such as spasticity, but the acceptance of spasticity as a concept and not as objective knowledge, together with the recommendation that a clinician using the term spasticity in a presentation or publication also provide the definition of spasticity held by that clinician, would be a good start and would facilitate discussion within the clinical society. It would also allow acceptance of different concepts and different therapeutic models; if two clinicians differ in their basic concepts then there is likely to be a corresponding difference in their therapeutic approach. This may raise concern regarding therapeutic relativism, where all therapeutic options are seen as valid, but is essentially a recognition of the present situation where there is considerable variation in clinical practice in terms of both clinical concepts and clinical management. Asking a clinician to explicitly state the concept upon which their therapeutic plan is based, and to provide evidence if available to support their approach, may help to clarify areas of agreement and variation between different approaches. This approach is discussed in more detail in Chapters 5 and 6. Ultimately, having a shared understanding of such terms as spasticity and having a shared expression of spasticity as an evolving concept or model rather than an objective entity would be ideal, but this may take some time.

Along with these steps it would be helpful for us to review our evidence base and to consider how we can make codified knowledge more available and more incorporated within our tacit knowledge. An increased understanding of statistics and data within the society in terms of sampling, data analysis, and data interpretation would be very helpful, as would an increased awareness of sources of bias in data interpretation. This is not intended as a criticism of bias as such as some bias, or context, is needed if any interpretation of data is to be made; what is needed instead is an awareness of the observer when we are considering the data. The resulting information then needs to be diffused within the society so that it moves from codified to tacit knowledge; there is, however, a concern that an increased awareness and understanding of the evidence available may improve our theoretical knowledge, but unless this information is transferrable to what Berger and Luckmann termed our 'pretheoretical knowledge', and becomes incorporated into 'what everyone knows', it is unlikely to influence overall clinical practice. The potential sources of bias in the evidence that we use to support our clinical practice are discussed in the next chapter, and our current approach to the formation of an evidence base is critically appraised in Chapter 5.

We will also need to consider how we learn from experience as clinicians and how we can use our experience and tacit knowledge to guide clinical management. As we discussed at the beginning of this chapter, acceptance of the validity of experience but also the limitations of experience is needed; in the words of Edmund Husserl, an Austrian philosopher, 'experience by itself is not science' (Husserl 1970). Husserl was concerned that when we come to a situation we bring prior conceptions about similar situations which influence our interpretation of the current situation. He encouraged us 'to see what stands before our eyes, to distinguish, to describe' and introduced the concept of 'bracketing', using the Greek word epoché, a term which was used by a philosophical school in Ancient Greece called the Sceptics to indicate a suspension of judgement. Husserl meant by bracketing or epoché that when we experience something we should strive to experience it directly, avoiding any preconceptions or ideas we may have, in a manner analogous to that advocated by Cage in his silent piece which we discussed earlier. An example of this in clinical practice could be the assessment of a child with cerebral palsy; rather than concluding on the basis of a clinical examination that the child has spasticity, we could instead describe what we have directly experienced. This could be a perception of resistance to passive movement of a joint, a perception of increased muscle activity, or a perception of reduced motor control. These findings will provide more specific information about the child than would be the case with the overall finding of 'spasticity'. In the same way, Husserl was keen that we rigorously describe the phenomena that we experience; this would mean defining how we make clinical measurements and how we ensure that these are valid and reliable. Although Husserl introduced these concepts almost 50 years before Polanyi wrote his book, Husserl's description of the need to be aware of our preconceptions can be interpreted in the light of Polanyi's concept of tacit knowledge. A clinical epoché would mean being conscious that our training and experience will influence our assessment and treatment of children with cerebral palsy and that our understanding of the underlying problem and our approach may not be shared by other clinicians with a different pattern of training and experience. This means that another clinician presented with the same clinical data may come to a different conclusion about the underlying problem and its management. Rather than trying to impose a uniform approach, if we work with other clinicians in a constructive manner to discuss the basis of our interpretation and of our clinical approach, this may allow us to clarify the concepts we share and clarify where we differ. This in turn may allow us to make our tacit or implicit knowledge explicit, and in this way facilitate discussion and understanding. Defining the concepts upon which we agree while accepting that different clinical approaches are valid because of our lack of information and uncertainty in the face of a complex clinical problem may be the most effective way to bring together different approaches in clinical management. This approach is discussed in more detail in Chapter 6.

THE OBJECTIVE BODY AND THE LIVED-IN BODY

Finally, we need to consider how our concepts regarding cerebral palsy and the management of musculoskeletal deformity relate to the lived experience of the child with cerebral palsy. This will be discussed in more detail in the final chapter but is worth considering briefly here as it allows for a shift in clinical approach, which can be helpful. Maurice Merleau-Ponty, the French philosopher mentioned above, studied the work of Husserl. Merleau-Ponty distinguished between what he termed the 'corps objectif', or objective body, and the 'corps propre', or lived-in and experiencing body (Merleau-Ponty 1962). The objective body is something that can be assessed and defined in anatomical, physiological, and pathological terms whereas the lived-in body is the first-person experience of the world by the child through their body.

The child with cerebral palsy will be aware of their body as themself; something 'lived-in' through which they experience life. Clinical practice, in contrast, may focus on the child's objective body; aspects that can be measured such as level of joint motion, level of deformity, muscle tone, and (depending on the definition of the observer) spasticity may be seen as important factors. A treatment approach aimed at assessing and treating an impairment such as spasticity may have an impact, whether positive or negative, on the child's objective body but may not have the same impact, or may have an unexpected impact, on the child's lived-in body. The quality of life of the child may be influenced by changes in their objective body but the effect of these will be mediated through the child's lived-in body in terms of whether pain, discomfort, or a limitation in function or participation is perceived by the child. Because of this, intervention to alter an impairment or an aspect of the objective body can only ever be a means to an end, namely a perception of improvement by the child in their experience of the world through their lived-in body. This could be achieved through the relief of pain, the maintenance or improvement of function, or through facilitation of participation or the development of interpersonal relationships.

Moving the focus of treatment from the child's objective body to their experience of the world through their lived-in body would have a number of positive consequences. Our concepts regarding the objective body, including tone, spasticity, and deformity, would need to be viewed in light of their relevance to the lived-in body. An intervention which alters an impairment without significantly altering the experience of life through their lived-in body would not be of value to the child. It is possible that when viewed in this way that some interventions currently performed may appear to be of more benefit to the clinician and the parents than to the child. A shift in focus to an approach centred on the daily experience of the child would be challenging but would offer the opportunity to place all of our interventions in perspective and to bring a unified theme to clinical management. We will discuss this further in Chapter 6.

In the next few chapters, we will look at how we obtain and interpret evidence to guide our clinical management. We will discuss how the musculoskeletal system may be more effectively viewed as a complex adaptive system rather than primarily as a structure, and we will review our current understanding of musculoskeletal growth and development in the typically developing child and discuss how this may be altered in children and young people with cerebral palsy. We will discuss how the evidence we use is based on the outcome of clinical studies in heterogenous groups, and discuss how to consider intervention for the individual based on evidence gained from the population. We will then look at how we can view our incomplete understanding of the complexity involved, and the associated uncertainty this implies for clinical management, in a positive light through a focus on the child's lived experience. The reader will be aware that as authors we will have our own preconceptions and biases, but hopefully our awareness of this will help us to maintain a viewpoint which at least aspires to objectivity. We do not underestimate the magnitude of the task ahead; encouraging an established clinical society to review and change some of its core concepts will be a challenge. On a positive note, the clinical society involved in the care of children with cerebral palsy is formed of committed and dedicated clinicians who are keen to provide the best possible care to the children they see.

A Made-Up Story About Data, Knowledge, and Clinical Judgement

A double-blind randomised controlled trial (RCT) has been conducted of an injectable pharmaceutical therapy (Zenetec) in a group of children with cerebral palsy between the ages of 6 and 11 years by an experienced group of clinician–researchers who have maintained an interest in this treatment through a history of case–control and cohort studies. The researchers on the RaSP-CP (Reducing SPasticity in Cerebral Palsy) trial recruited 60 participants (30 to the intervention arm and 30 to the control [no treatment arm]). Sammi, Kamal, and Beth all participated in the trial. Twelve weeks after the injections, the researchers found significant effects in the domains of functional capacity (Gross Motor Function Measure-66; GMFM-66) and performance (Canadian Occupational Performance Measure; COPM), while there have been non-significant findings in a measure of participation (Life-H) and in the level of contentment of the parents of the children. Six months later, there were no significant differences. They conclude that the trial demonstrated that the pharmaceutical therapy is effective for the short-term management of spasticity. Dr Plum (lead investigator) submits the manuscript to a leading journal on behalf of all the authors. The article was reviewed by five blinded reviewers drawn from academics and clinicians well known in the area. There was some difference of opinion between the reviewers but the associate editor to which the article was allocated decides to go with the majority view, and with some minor modifications, the article is published.

New knowledge can be created from a well-conducted and considered trial of a new type of physiotherapy programme, novel medicinal product, or modified surgical method.

A panel of experts recruited by a governmental quango to provide guidance to clinicians on treatments in spastic cerebral palsy has reported its considerations. The expert panel is composed of leading clinicians in the management of spasticity in cerebral palsy, and supported by specialists in assessing evidence and in quality assurance. The expert clinicians know each other well, having worked on similar panels before and worked with each other on collaborative research projects. Many of them also know and respect the lead researcher in the team who has reported their research on the new pharmaceutical, Zenetec. A number have conducted similar trials to the one above. They decide on the back of the article above and by other recent articles in the literature to support the clinical use of Zenetec and similar therapies for children up to 11 years of age.

Advancement of care for a group of individuals with cerebral palsy is dependent on translating valid knowledge from research studies into clinical care guidelines.

A young paediatrician, Dr Jenny Jackson, with a few years of experience in directing treatment in children, has read the recently published guideline. In her clinic this morning, she has Joe, a young person of 11 years with a diagnosis of spastic cerebral palsy. She talks to the family about the new guidance from the expert panel, and strongly suggests that the family consider the new medicine. Overall, the family are receptive to the young doctor's enthusiasm, but they have been here before. A few years ago, Joe had tried an oral medication, and didn't get on with it. Later, Dr Jackson meets her senior colleague, and talks to her about the case. Dr Esther Akinluyi knows the family well and recalls Joe's adverse reaction to the previous medication. Esther advises Jenny to proceed cautiously. She suggests that the team gather more experience of the new treatment in those who fit more closely the characteristics of the participants in the study.

Sound clinical judgment and decision-making requires interpreting the available research and its derivative guidelines carefully in the context of the individual's physical, behavioural, and cognitive characteristics, their circumstances, and their preferences.

Dr Jackson meets with the family again and they agree to go ahead with the treatment. Dr Jackson informs Andrew Sellers, Joe's new physiotherapist, of the forthcoming intervention so that Andrew can spot any alteration in Joe's spasticity and function over the next few months. Andrew is enthusiastic about the prospect of the new treatment, and of meeting Joe. At Joe's first appointment with Andrew, Andrew assesses Joe with the Modified Tardieu Scale (MTS) and performs the GMFM. The MTS score at the first assessment is quite high. Andrew hopes that the new treatment will have a positive effect, and reassures Joe that he thinks that it will. Joe receives the treatment during the following week. When Andrew sees Joe again, 3 months later, Andrew's measurement of Joe's spasticity on the MTS is reduced by a point and his GMFM has gone up a couple of points. Joe reports that he is feeling tired and weak, but everybody is happy that the treatment appears to be working.

Many of the treatments carried out in children and adults with cerebral palsy are short-term and require comprehensive evaluation. Assessment of the individual's response to treatment depends on the clinician's interpretation of measurements made on that individual before and after intervention and to the trajectory of that individual's natural history.

In Chapter 1, we reflected on the nature of knowledge in clinical science. In this chapter, we will discuss how clinical knowledge is created and applied, through the vehicle of the 'made-up' story above. We will consider the weaknesses of evidence-based medicine as it is currently practiced, particularly RCTs. We will look at how we interpret research findings both as authors and readers, and how we might improve the transfer of knowledge between the researcher and the clinician to benefit patients. Then, our attention will turn to the synthesis of evidence to inform guidelines on the management of cerebral palsy. We will look at the methodology, and the composition of the expert panel, used to produce a guideline. The application of guidelines in clinical practice and the conversation between clinician, parent, and patient will be discussed. We will dedicate some pages to the nature of clinical observations (measurements) made on the patient and whether those observations, or changes in them, should be considered significant. In the later pages of this chapter, we will draw together some of the conclusions of these arguments. In some ways, this chapter is about our (researchers, clinicians, and patients) relationship with numbers.

How numbers are used to determine the initial course of treatment and how they are used to maintain or terminate it.

THE RANDOMISED CONTROLLED TRIAL

The 'criterion standard' of modern prospective clinical research is the RCT. Although regulated clinical trials have existed since the second half of the 19th century, the first successful RCT in medicine was introduced in 1948 by a team involving Austin Bradford Hill, a British epidemiologist (Marshall et al. 1948). The Medical Research Council sponsored investigators team assessed the effectiveness of Streptomycin in the management of pulmonary disease.

Initially, RCTs were not welcomed warmly by the pharmaceutical industry. But, after the Thalidomide scandal in the early 1960s, US Congress introduced legislation that demanded 'adequate and well-controlled investigations' of drugs before approval (Greene and Podolsky 2012). By the early 1970s, the Food and Drug Administration (FDA) interpreted Congress' requirement as the provision of evidence from RCTs. Many of the early trials were very successful because they were able to show clear benefits of a new treatment against a placebo (indeed, the Streptomycin trial was strongly positive in comparison to bedrest). However, RCTs work less well in the area of paediatric neurodisability because it is difficult to meet three important conditions: (1) an adequate sample size in the face of a target population which is characterised by variation in severity and phenotype; (2) removal of the significant sources of bias; and (3) measurements of long-term responses to the treatment in individuals undergoing significant development.

In the context of the medicine that Joe is taking. The RCT conducted appears to be well controlled but let us look at the story behind the article in the literature. Would this trial meet the conditions set out above?

SAMPLE SIZES AND OUTCOME STATISTICS IN RANDOMISED CONTROLLED TRIALS

The variation in location, timing, and extent of the cerebral injury in cerebral palsy gives rise to diverse clinical presentations with different levels of severity and anatomical distribution of involvement, as well as varied neurological features, and frequent comorbidities. All the children were included in the featured clinical trial because they had a diagnosis of spastic cerebral palsy and had increased tone (as measured in their lower limbs by the Modified Ashworth Scale) at two or more joint levels (Fosang et al. 2003). However, individual children within the trial differed greatly. Sammi, for example, has epilepsy, has greater involvement of his upper limbs than either Kamal or Beth, and he met his motor milestones at a greater age than his two coparticipants.

Although one of the inclusion criteria for the study was that the child must be able to walk independently or with assistance, Sammi uses a posterior walker, and then only on rare occasions. Mostly, Sammi uses his wheelchair for mobility. Kamal walks well

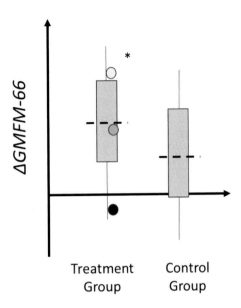

Figure 2.1 The results of the RaSP-CP trial in the functional capacity domain are depicted. The specific results for Sammi (black circle), Kamal (mid-grey circle), and Beth (light-grey circle) are depicted.

independently but has an asymmetric presentation and has some difficulties understanding instruction. Beth has mild restrictions in passive range and high tone. Figure 2.1 shows the changes in gross motor function (GMFM-66) across the 60 participants in both the treatment and control arms of the study. The result is significant. The participants in the treatment group fair better in the GMFM-66 domains and in aspects of functional performance (COPM) as indicated by a p-value of less than 0.05.

From Figure 2.1, we can see that Beth, Sammi, and Kamal have varied responses within a group that, in itself, shows diverse responses. The results for these individuals beg some interesting questions. Is Beth's positive outcome secondary to a reduction in her tone due to the action of the pharmaceutical? Is Sammi's more negative response related to underlying weakness? In other words, are there specific characteristics of the individual patients within the group of participants which predispose them to a beneficial (or poor) response to the treatment or are the results of the study independent of the particular characteristics of Sammi, Kamal, or Beth, and are due, say, to the intrinsic errors of the measurement methodologies employed? The truth is that for this hypothetical trial, and for many other real trials of a similar nature (see Chapter 4), one cannot tell.

For a clinician to be confident that the results of a simple comparative trial (such as the RaSP-CP trial) are relevant to the child in front of them, the results of the study must be 'convincing', that is, that substantially more of the participants show a more positive response in the treatment arm than the control arm.

There are statistics that we could apply to the results from RCTs to quantify 'convincing'. In 1992, Jacob Cohen described a simple dimensionless statistic which summarises

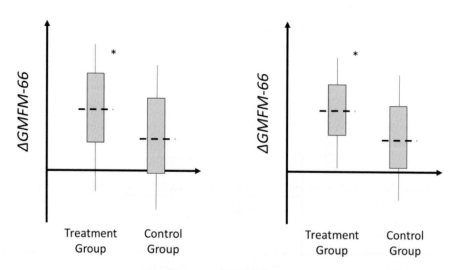

Figure 2.2 The data from the RaSP-CP trial is featured. A further fictitious data set is also shown where the variation response in the treatment group is lower.

the effect size of the results from a trial (Cohen 1992). Cohen's *d* (sometimes called the standardised effect size) is the ratio of the mean response to a measure of the spread of the responses, in this case, a measure of the pooled standard deviation of the samples (Equation 2.1).

$$\text{Cohen's d} = \frac{\textit{Mean treatment group} - \textit{Mean control group}}{\textit{Pooled standard devitation}}$$

Equation 2.1

Let's apply Cohen's *d* to the results of our hypothetical trial and an alternative data set that we have just made up! For Cohen's *d* an effect size of 0.2 to 0.3 is considered to be a 'small' effect, around 0.5 a 'medium' effect, and 0.8 to infinity a 'large' effect.

In Figure 2.2, both studies give rise to a significant difference (a *p*-value less than 0.05, that is, a likelihood of less than one in 20 that the null hypothesis, that there is no statistical difference between treatment and control, is correct). The values of Cohen's *d* in each study are different with the higher value in our alternative data set. This is because the spread of data in the treatment group is lower, resulting in a smaller value of the pooled standard deviation (Equation 2.1). A higher Cohen's *d* is indicative of a more successful trial specifically that there is a greater likelihood of a positive outcome for any individual patient that would fit the inclusion and exclusion criteria of the trial. So why is Cohen's *d* or similar measures of effect size (such as standardised mean difference) not more widely quoted in the literature in trials in cerebral palsy, when they are readily calculable? First, we must consider what researchers think RCTs are for. The scientific method demands that we prove an original hypothesis (or disprove a null hypothesis). In this way, RCTs are often successful because they calculate *p*-values. We could say that RCTs have *internal validity*, that is, they do what they are supposed to do, normally prove there is an independent interaction between an intervention and the change in an outcome measure. Second, many of the trials in cerebral palsy would produce effect sizes that were considered small or medium, so it is not in the academic interests of the researchers to quote them (it would make the trial seem less successful). Third, Cohen's *d* is a largely unintuitive statistic. What do 'small', 'medium', and 'large' effect sizes really mean and how would a clinician use them in a consultation to explain the likely benefit and risks of treatment to their patient or to the patient's parents?

In the case of the RaSP-CP trial, how could its design, execution, and reporting have been improved, so that the response to treatment of patients similar to Sammi, Kamal, and Beth might be better predicted by their clinicians?

Before the researchers in the RaSP-CP trial conducted their experiments, they performed a sample size calculation. The purpose of the calculation is to estimate the numbers of participants required to reduce two types of error. The first type is the likelihood of disproving the null hypothesis incorrectly (known as a type I error) and the second is the likelihood of supporting a false null hypothesis (known as a type II error). The only way to reduce type I *and* II errors is to increase the sample size. In this case, the type I error is the likelihood of showing the response to the pharmaceutical was positive when it was not and the type II error would have been to show that the response to the pharmaceutical was not positive, when in fact, it was. Using data from their previous cohort studies, the researchers estimated that they needed 30 participants in each arm of the trial in order to reduce the chance of a type I error to 5% and the chance of a type II error to 10%. As you might surmise, the size of a sample is estimated according to the overall (mean) response in the trial, and according to their simple hypothesis.

Most trials in cerebral palsy have sample sizes that have been estimated according to simple hypotheses, just like in the RaSP-CP trial and, in general, the numbers are not large enough to confidently perform subgroup analyses (on, e.g. sex or phenotype) or regression analysis against the potential covariates (such as body mass, age, and severity of 'spasticity'). The RaSP-CP trial is not designed to tell us about potentially important characteristics of Sammi, Kamal, and Beth that might influence their response to the pharmaceutical.

How could we make results of research studies more relevant to individual patients? One possible solution is to narrow the inclusion criteria to a group of participants where the researchers are more confident that there is likely to be a benefit – perhaps, they have conducted some previous exploratory work, the results of which suggest that a subgroup of the sample population, that have similar characteristics to Beth, may respond more profitably, that is, have a greater Cohen's *d* value. The problem is that such a trial would clearly lack generalisability (the applicability of the results to a broad range of patients), and it may be difficult to recruit adequate numbers of children who 'look' like Beth, which would reduce the likelihood of a significant result. Multicentre trials have the potential to recruit greater numbers of participants (so that subgroup analysis and regressions may be performed) but there are logistical and methodological barriers to success. Multicentre trials are expensive to conduct, difficult to organise, and require a degree of conformity in practice across centres (Brown, Bachmann, and Foster 2013). There are very few multicentre trials in cerebral palsy. Even in these rare cases, a statistical explanation of the variation in the response of individuals within the group tends to be missing.

Are there alternatives to RCTs? The improvements in computing power and algorithm development allow alternative investigations of real-world clinical data that may help us to fit the patient to the best existing treatment. This works by forming large databases collated from the data of individual centres that use similar forms of patient assessment, treatments, and outcome measures. 'Real-world' here means that we use existing clinical data and accept small amounts of variation in practice across practitioners, and contributing institutions. Powerful statistical methods (such as decision trees or naïve Bayesian methods) are used to calculate the probability of success of a specific treatment from large pools of historic data, and help the individual clinician to decide on the course of management. In some areas of paediatrics, the method has been shown to improve clinical outcomes in terms of higher survival rates and reduction of adverse effects (Kokol, Završnik, and Vošner 2017). Even in cerebral palsy, some institutions have large enough databases to develop tools to predict outcome from a specific orthopaedic surgery according to the individual characteristics of the patient (Schwartz et al. 2013). Criticisms of a big data approach to clinical decision support and to research would include the same criticisms of large observational studies such as bias and lack of explanation of causal relationships (mechanisms of disease progression and of intervention). Database studies are necessarily limited to retrospective studies of existing practice, so perhaps the biggest criticism of these approaches comes from the lack of creation of new scientific knowledge. For example, if a researcher is trying a radically new surgical intervention they would *have to* conduct a prospective study. On the other hand, a database study of an existing surgical method may be considered a good alternative to an RCT where there are considerable methodological, logistical, and ethical problems to successful completion.

The second reason for the lack of reporting of effect sizes in published research in musculoskeletal management in cerebral palsy is that, often, they are not very impressive! In the RaSP-CP trial, a Cohen's *d* of 0.33, which is considered 'small', could have been reported by the authors but was not. The authors know very well the bias that exists in the publication of positive and negative results, and they have invested a lot of effort in conducting the study. The lead researcher is ambitious for an academic promotion to a personal chair. The publication of an RCT and the funding that might follow would certainly support that application. It is not in the interests of a clinical researcher or team of researchers to report moderate effect sizes.

Although Cohen suggested a convention by which the magnitude of effect sizes might be judged, the third reason why Cohen's *d* is not reported is that the number does not have a meaning that is relevant to the clinical practitioner. Thankfully, there are alternatives to Cohen's *d* used in medicine that are more intuitive, and would be helpful to the clinician to explain if the treatment is more or less likely to benefit their patient. Relative risk (RR) is the probability of improvement (or worsening) in the treatment group divided by the probability of improvement (or worsening) in the control (placebo) group (Table 2.1 and Equation 2.2).

$$\textit{Relative Risk (RR)} = \frac{w}{w+y} \div \frac{x}{x+z} \qquad\qquad \textit{Equation 2.2}$$

$$\textit{Odds Ratio (OR)} = \frac{w}{y} \div \frac{x}{z} \qquad\qquad \textit{Equation 2.3}$$

Table 2.1. Numbers of participants in a trial allocated according to whether they improved or declined according to the outcome measure used

	Better than neutral	Worse than neutral
Intervention	W	Y
Control	X	Z

The RR is an easy statistic to understand. A value of 1 means that the treatment is as likely as the control to result in a benefit, whereas a value of 2 indicates the treatment is twice as likely. The odds ratio (OR) is only slightly more complicated. It is the proportion of participants improved in the treatment group divided by the proportion of participants improved in the control group. If we analysed the results from the GMFM-66 in the RaSP-CP trial presented in Figure 1.2, RR has a value of 10/9 indicating that the probability of benefitting from the treatment is only a little more than benefitting from the control. OR has a value of 5/3 indicating that the odds of benefitting over worsening is 1.667 time greater in the treatment group than in the control group. Publication of statistics such as OR and RR might facilitate a different sort of conversation with Dr Jenny Jackson's patient, Joe. Instead of saying that this treatment has been shown to work (because it has a p-value of less than 0.05) she would have been able to say to Joe that your chances of improving are just a little better than if we did nothing or (if Joe was betting man) your odds are 5/3 times better if you select the treatment. Perhaps these numbers may have even caused Dr Jackson some reflection.

Let's extend this idea of knowledge transfer by creating some statistics with even more utility than OR or RR. Even if a trial had very favourable values for these statistics, it would not tell us what the chances were of our patient improving or deteriorating by a *meaningful* amount. It is quite possible that all the participants in the treatment arm of a study improve in terms of the outcome variable but none of them actually feel better. We could improve upon RR and OR with a statistic based on the concept of minimal clinically important difference (MCID). An MCID is the smallest difference in a variable thought to represent a real benefit (or deterioration) to the patient in terms of their quality of life, their participation, or their own perception of wellness. There are three ways that an MCID can be estimated (Cook 2008). There are methods based on the distribution of the outcome data (called distribution methods). These have been criticised in the academic literature because they are not referenced to a clinician's or patient's subjective understanding of change. Alternatively, a group of experts can decide by a system called the Delphi method. The Delphi method is an iterative process in which experts decide what constitutes a meaningful outcome. The third method is where the MCID is anchored to the patients' (or their representatives') subjective views of being better or worse. Each method has its weaknesses, but perhaps the biggest issue in physical disability is that the calculation of MCID is rare by any method.

Let us consider the likely impact application of this simple concept would have on the interpretation of our hypothetical RaSP-CP trial. The MCID for the GMFM-66 has been estimated at about 2.7 points (Oeffinger et al. 2008). Figure 2.3 illustrates the number of individuals who would have improved by a clinically significant amount, worsened by a

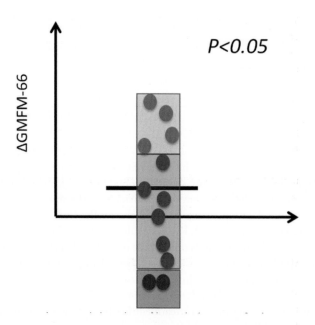

Figure 2.3 Changes in Gross Motor Function Measure (GMFM) after treatment in an intervention arm. The lighter shaded area represents participants who have improved by more than a minimal clinically important difference (MCID). The darker shaded area represents those who have deteriorated by more than an MCID. The middle shaded area represents those participants who have not changed by an MCID.

clinically significant amount, or did not change by a clinically significant amount. We can form a table containing these numbers (Table 2.2) and develop simple statistics as follows:

Table 2.2 Numbers of participants in a study demonstrating clinically significant improvement, no change, or a significant worsening

	Clinically significant improvement	No clinically significant change	Clinically significant decline
Intervention	P	Q	R
Control	S	T	U

In the treatment arm of the study, we can estimate the chance of improving by simply calculating the ratio of those in the study who benefitted by more than an MCID to the total participants in the study. Similarly, we can calculate the chance of worsening by more than the MCID (see Equations 2.4 and 2.5 below).

$$probClinicalBenefit = \frac{p}{p + q + r} \qquad \text{Equation 2.4}$$

$$probClinicalRisk = \frac{r}{p + q + r} \qquad \text{Equation 2.5}$$

Equations 2.4 and 2.5 describe simple statistics indicating risk and benefit in a single arm of a simple comparative trial.

One can create similar probabilities indicating ratio of likelihoods of clinically significant improvement in the treatment and control groups. In any case, Dr Jenny Jackson may now have an even more interesting conversation with Joe and his parents. 'Our best research in this area suggests that if you choose this intervention you have a one in three chance of getting better, you have a one in six chance of getting worse and you have a 50% chance of staying where you are.' With information like this, Joe and his family can weigh their own personal preferences against the probabilities of success and failure, and take an active part in the decision-making. For example, Joe may be deeply unhappy with his present situation, and the prospect of improvement, even if it has a low probability, may seem like a risk worth taking. On the other hand, Joe might be reasonably content, and consider the risk of decline, even if it has a low probability, not worthwhile.

BIAS IN RANDOMISED CONTROLLED TRIALS

One of the reasons to conduct an RCT, as opposed to a cohort study or a non-randomised trial, is to reduce possible bias in the design of the study, recruitment of participants, and the generation and reporting of results. However, even RCTs are not free from bias. Here, we will discuss the sources of bias that affect, in particular, trials in musculoskeletal treatments in children and adults with cerebral palsy. We will use the RaSP-CP trial to illustrate some of these potential biases, and propose some solutions.

In our hypothetical trial, the investigators decided to compare their new treatment against a placebo control. Any significant result here would mean, in general, that the intervention is better than doing nothing. But what about all the treatments that have a reported positive effect on spasticity? Surely, the authors should be comparing with these, more proven, interventions. The bias here is in the design of the trial.

Double-blinded RCTs are considered among the most important original sources of evidence in the world of clinical research. Blinding reduces *ascertainment bias*, that is the bias introduced by the investigators and/or the participants having knowledge of the assignment of the participants during the intervention(s). The alternative to a blinded study is an 'open-label' trial in which the participants and investigators are aware of the assignment of participants. Research suggests that open-label trials may exaggerate treatment effects positively by 17% (Schulz et al. 1995) compared to double-blinded trials.

Some types of study are hard to blind. Take, for example, studies of short-term stretch-casting. Participants will always know if they have been cast or not! Investigators will probably know because of any marks left on the limb by the cast or by communication with the participant. Surgery is also very hard to blind. Some surgical studies have attempted to blind patients and investigators by introducing a sham surgery in the placebo group. This may be considered unethical and there have not been any sham surgical studies reported in children with cerebral palsy.

The RaSP-CP trial was reported to be double-blinded. Vials containing the active drug or saline were given to the investigators after random allocation of the participants. This would seem like an effective way of blinding the investigators and the participants.

However, the drug under investigation has a 'distinctive' side-effect, a transient weakness of the muscle group into which it has been injected. Those who witnessed this, or those who were told about it second-hand, would have known that the child had been allocated to the treatment group. If a 'believer' in this medication was aware, their behaviours might be affected: the way they approach the child during a clinical history or any other subjective assessment, or the encouragement of the child during a physical therapy session. If the parents were aware of this drug's side-effects, they may have filled out the Life-H questionnaire more positively. Dr Plum, seeing a poor result from a participant in the treatment group, may find a reason to omit it. The point here is that it is very hard to truly blind those involved in trials, even those trials that are reported to be blinded.

The inability to blind certain types of study introduces its own sort of bias. The purpose of systematic reviews and meta-analyses is to indicate the strength of evidence to support or negate an intervention (Wilt and Fink 2007). Unblinded trials have less evidential weight in these reviews. Consequently, trials involving surgeries or casting may not reach the levels of support within meta-analyses that say a pharmaceutical therapy receives.

Some biases are subtle but may have a powerful influence on the outcome of the study. Becky, a junior member of Dr Plum's team, is recruiting patients and allocating them according to the agreed randomisation procedure. Having been part of the research team for a couple of years, she has become familiar with how Dr Plum thinks. She knows that he believes that there will be an interaction between severity of the patients' levels of spasticity as measured by the Tardieu Scale and the effect of the treatment. Becky is supposed to recruit according to the stated inclusion and exclusion criteria but because she is aware of a possible interaction, she applies them in such a way to exclude several individuals with relatively low scores on the Modified Tardieu Scale that should have properly been included in the study. Her bias at recruitment means that the trial becomes less generalisable to the population, and, if she guessed right and there was a real interaction between Modified Tardieu Scale and the intervention, she would have affected the results in favour of the treatment.

Biases can occur right through the development of a piece of research from conception to reporting. Most clinical trials are funded by a national or international charity or state-supported non-governmental organisation. These organisations have research agendas set out by senior members of the medical and scientific community. The members of the panels that sit on the scientific advisory committees of these institutions, and the reviewers that score the grant applications, are executors of the policies of the charitable or governmental institution. Additionally, these individuals may have models in their heads of how a study should be designed and what questions the application should be seeking the answer to. Experienced and successful researchers, like Dr Plum, sit on these panels and so understand the zeitgeist and know which boxes to tick. Consequently, prospective research is influenced heavily by the current agreed view created by those who are often the recipients of the awards.

Biases also happen during the process of manuscript authoring. Old heads, like Dr Plum, know how to promote certain results within the set of results that have been produced by the study. We do not want to pick out Dr Plum for particular scrutiny; in nearly all the research articles you will read in the area of cerebral palsy, the authors will select the one or two positive results from the many results that were insignificant. In Dr Plum's case, the emphasis he placed on the improvements in GMFM and COPM disguised the less impressive results for participation and parental satisfaction, and he was able to state in his conclusive paragraph that:

> In a double-blind randomised sham-controlled trial, intramuscular injections of Zenetec and therapy were effective for improving motor capacity and motor performance in ambulant children with cerebral palsy.

One can reduce allocation, assignment, and reporting biases by putting protocols in place that reduce the likelihood of the investigators guessing to which group the participants or the data belongs. These might include making the roles of the investigators distinct from each other, such as differentiating the roles of recruitment and allocation, and of assessment and data analysis. The bias introduced by Dr Plum's interpretation of the results could be minimised if the data analysts in his team presented him with results in which the intervention and control groups were masked.

Bias is often a process that happens in the subconscious, and we are not suggesting that all researchers are cheats. However, we should be aware of the potential biases of research studies when reading research articles. It would be helpful if the editors of journals insisted that researchers explained in more detail in a supplement to their main paper about their strategies to reduce bias in their studies. This would make researchers more vigilant and give the readership more confidence.

SHORT-TERM FOLLOW-UP AND LONG-TERM OUTCOMES

Children with cerebral palsy have a life-long neuromuscular condition for which there is no cure. Management options are limited to alleviating the symptoms of the underlying problems to improve or maintain mobility, participation, and communication over the lifespan. These children also have accompanying conditions which may affect their neuromuscular condition and its management such as malnutrition, epilepsy, and visual problems. RCTs and, indeed, other sorts of interventional studies in cerebral palsy, focus on short-term goals (between weeks and a year typically). We should question whether short-term results are always relevant to our long-term objectives. Let us again turn to the RaSP-CP trial as an example to illustrate the point. The pharmaceutical therapy is delivered to target muscles with the aim of reducing the effects of abnormal muscle activation on the quality of movement thus improving motor control. Zenetec interferes with the release of acetylcholine into the neuromuscular junction and prevents muscle activation. The results presented in the paper are from 12 weeks and 6 months after injection. At 6 months, there were no significant results. Does this mean the clinician in charge of the patient should be happy to reinject periodically to maintain the moderate short-term benefits that may be offered by the intervention? There are two main factors to consider. First, the children recruited to the RaSP-CP trial were Zenetec naïve. There could be an interaction between the number of previous injections and the effectiveness of any new injection, so, as they stand, the results from the trial do not support Zenetec as an on-going therapy. Second, muscles develop in size and composition rapidly during childhood to maintain movement function despite great increases in body mass. The effect of Zenetec on muscle development was not investigated in the RaSP-CP trial and therefore we do not know of the long-term effects of the therapy on gross motor function, but if it did interfere with muscle development, the child may be left with an unwanted legacy when they are older.

In the absence of high quality long-term data, it is important that the clinician charged with the care of children with cerebral palsy understands the mechanisms of action of the interventions that they might consider, so that they can assure themselves that an adverse long-term interaction of their intervention and natural history is unlikely.

CLINICAL GUIDELINES

The RCT performed by Dr Plum and his colleagues was reviewed by a panel of experts on behalf of a national organisation responsible for the creation of clinical management guidelines. Many countries have independent non-governmental bodies like the National Council for Clinical Advice (NCCA) that provide guidelines on clinical management. The institution makes recommendations for public health and health care technology assessment, as well as clinical guidelines for managing clinical problems. Clinical guideline development teams consist of different stakeholders including experts, practitioners, specialists in systematic review and in quality assurance, as well as members of the public. Where possible the panel are required to consider the evidence for assessments and interventions both in terms of clinical efficacy and cost. There is little doubt that many of the guidelines produced by NCCA have had a very positive impact on clinical care. For example, 14 years ago, they produced a guideline for the early management of head injuries in adults, recommending that computed tomography scans were used in all cases for the detection of intracranial hematoma. The clinical guideline was based on considerable evidence in the literature and the panel were happy that computed tomography would pick up nearly 100% of the hematomas present and had reasonable specificity. This is a powerful example of a good clinical guideline. Variation in practice existed before the implementation of the guideline. The clinical guideline group implemented a guideline based on *very* strong evidence, and were able to unify clinical practice. Some years later, a similar guideline was produced for head injury management in paediatrics.

One of the teams recruited by NCCA reviewed the evidence for treatments of spasticity in children with a focus on cerebral palsy. Among many other articles, the team reviewed the work of Dr Plum and his team on Zenetec and works of other research groups on competitive spasticity management medications, as well as alternative therapies such as physiotherapy and surgery. The team may have recognised that the quantity and quality of evidence supporting Zenetec and other treatments like it are thin. They may have, like we have, noticed that the effect sizes for these interventions are poor. They may have even spotted that the methodology applied is weak. However, they have been instructed by the NCCA to discuss a set of recommendations for these treatments. How did they proceed, and how might they have proceeded?

In fact, the clinical guideline development group could not make a definitive statement. They recommended that 'injectable spasticity therapies (such as Zenetec) be considered for clinical use, taking into account patient preferences, particular characteristics of the patient etc'. The statement is vague but positively accented. Instead, they could have easily written that

> clinicians should be cautious when considering these therapies owing to the heterogeneity in the response of individuals with cerebral palsy and the moderate mean treatment effect. At the present time, we do not know which characteristics of the individual with spastic cerebral palsy would predict a successful response to the therapy, or, equally, predict a negative one.

Why did the panel opt for the more positive option with non-committal language?

In Chapter 1, we contemplated the idea of the clinical science society. It is important to most individuals within a group to maintain harmony of the group. This need to be in harmony is explained by a concept offered by evolutionary anthropologists in which the successful maintenance of the tribal society relies upon consensus of the individuals making up that community. For the tribal society to continue, deviants to the consensus view (the status quo) need to be removed or marginalised. The clinical membership of clinical guidance panels tends to consist of individuals who, in general, know each other, and who belong to a broader clinical community. The members of the spasticity management guideline development group are users of spasticity management medication similar to Zenetec. Individual panellists may be programmed to support the functioning of the panel rather than enter contentious discussions about one treatment or other, marking themselves out as a maverick and endangering their own position within the panel, and within their own clinical community. The wording of the final recommendations of the panel may reflect as much the need to maintain the status quo as to challenge it.

In the Clinic

In a delightful article in the *BMJ* some years ago, Isaacs and Fitzgerald proposed that doctors were highly influenced by their peers suggesting that eminence is more influential than evidence in guiding clinical practice (Isaacs and Fitzgerald 1999). There is often a nugget of truth in a comic observation. Hospital doctors, physiotherapists, and primary care practitioners do not, in general, read the academic literature (Barraclough 2004). Rather, they form their views on assessment and treatment from the opinion-makers in their midst, from their own experience, and from clinical guidelines. Dr Jenny Jackson is a recently qualified paediatrician. Reviewing children with cerebral palsy for their physical management takes up only 5% of her time. Jenny is a keen follower of the NCCA guidelines, having used them previously in the management of asthma and eczema, and assessment for bacterial meningitis.

Today, Jenny is seeing Joe in her clinic. Joe is an 11-year-old boy with spastic cerebral palsy. Joe has been coming to the community clinic since his diagnosis 8 and a half years ago, but his care has been transferred to Jenny from Dr Esther Akinluyi, the senior paediatrician at the clinic. Jenny knows that Esther likes to manage children like Joe very conservatively. Jenny reviews Joe's medical record briefly before the arrival of Joe and his family. She notes that Joe is independently ambulant and doing well at school, and that his treatment in recent times has been limited to an exercise programme that has been reviewed monthly.

From her reading, she forms the opinion that Joe's family believe that Joe's mobility has been stable over the last year but that they are open to discussing alternative interventions. She goes to the NCCA website and looks for guidance. She finds the clinical guidance on spasticity management and reads the recommendations. Joe seems to fit the criteria for injectable spasticity medication of which Zenetec is one popular branded form.

At the clinic appointment, Jenny proposes that the family considers the therapy. They seem a little reluctant, but Jenny prints out some information, and asks them to return in a few weeks. Later that day, Jenny discusses Joe with Esther. Esther is concerned that Jenny is advancing Joe's care a little too quickly. She remembers that Joe had some mild side-effects when he was put on a previous oral medication to reduce his tone. Jenny doesn't say much, but she thinks that Esther is too concerned about any side-effects from Zenetec and doesn't believe that there is a relationship between the two therapies. Joe, and his mother and father, really like Jenny, and they respond to her positivity. At the next appointment, the family agree to trying the therapy and Jenny sends a referral to a paediatrician that she knows who does the injections. She also refers Joe to Andrew Sellers, a physiotherapist in the practice, for a pre-assessment of Joe's range of motion and mobility.

It is useful to take a critical look at Jenny's decision-making. First, Jenny did not access data that might have helped her evaluate competitive therapies for Joe. If she had read Dr Plum's paper, she may have noticed that the difference between the mean change in the treatment and control group was not large and that the standard deviations associated with the mean change in the treatment group were wide, suggesting a good deal of heterogeneity in response to the therapy. She would have seen that Joe was at the top end of the age range in the study, which may have implied that he would be less responsive. She could have communicated these results and the results from alternative treatments to the parents and to Joe. That way, and second, she could have entered into a wider-ranging discussion about intervention incorporating risks and benefits, parental and patient preferences, and their goals. Finally, there was no rush. In general, decisions over physical management in cerebral palsy do not need to be taken in haste. Spending one or two consultations developing a relationship with the family may have served Joe's long-term needs better than looking for a quick fix.

Measuring Outcomes

When conducting a clinical interview with a patient or reading the medical notes, one often notices that a medication or other therapy has been continued for some time without comprehensive re-evaluation. Other times, treatment has been discontinued without a clear rationale or a proper assessment of the patient's status. How should we decide to continue or stop treatment to a patient once a treatment has been initiated?

Measuring outcome is an essential element of any interventional research study. Dr Plum and his team chose to measure gross motor function (GMFM-66) and functional performance (COPM) because changes in these variables are considered important to the patient. In the Zenetec trial, we know that there was a central tendency for the GMFM-66 and the COPM to improve in the short term but that in many individual participants these variables seemingly worsened. The difference between the central tendency and an individual's measured response to a medication may be due to the characteristics of the individual, inconsistency in the delivery of the treatment, or to errors in the measurement of the variable. For the individual patient, evaluating outcome means making objective and subjective measurements of their status to establish if their condition has truly improved, deteriorated, or stayed the same. Measuring outcome is a cornerstone of good clinical practice because it personalises the evidence for an intervention. The decision to initiate a treatment may have been based on the available published clinical guidance and the relevant characteristics of the patient, but the decision to repeat a treatment should be based on the individual's response to that treatment. Close monitoring of the patient's responses to any intervention is always desirable but particularly when there is less than compelling evidence to support the intervention in the first place. Jenny Jackson used Zenetec initially based largely on the advice of the NCCA. Wisely, she decided to evaluate Joe's function before the first injection and at 12 weeks after the injection. However, were the measurements taken a fair reflection of Joe's response to treatment?

The first step in evaluating outcome is deciding on the outcome measures to employ. Helpfully, the World Health Organization's International Classification of Functioning, Disability and Health (ICF) describes three contributing factors to disability – impairment, activity limitation, and participation restriction (https://www.who.int/classifications/icf/en/). The impairment in Joe's case is an abnormality in muscle activity which is interfering with his motor function. Joe's reduced motor capacity may be associated with his ability to kick a ball with power and accuracy, and so his participation in team sports may be restricted. Outcome measures should be selected that reflect broadly all aspects of the ICF. For Joe, only two (clinically reported) outcome measures have been adopted and these did not include measurements of activity limitation or participation.

Often, when we make a measurement of impairment, we do not directly quantify the underlying pathology but a symptom of it. The danger for any clinician or researcher is that they may begin to confuse the measurement with the pathology. Andrew Sellers, Joe's new physiotherapist, has been asked to use the Modified Tardieu Scale to assess Joe's level of spasticity. The Modified Tardieu Scale is a 5-point scale in which the rater rotates a joint rapidly and scores the resistance to movement from no resistance to an infatigable clonus (Boyd and Graham 1999). In the most commonly quoted definition, spasticity is defined as a motor disorder characterised by a velocity-dependent reflex (Lance 1980). Just because we see one of the symptoms of spasticity (the reflexive response) diminish after treatment we should not necessarily believe that the treatment has worked to reduce spasticity. Otherwise, an effective management option for managing spasticity would be a 'musculectomy' in which the offending muscle is removed. The component of the reflexive arc due to rapid stretching of that muscle is obliviated but so is much else! Andrew Sellers was happy that Joe had a reduced score on the Modified Tardieu Scale after treatment, but was Joe's spasticity really managed or, simply, was the potential of the muscle to generate force reduced? We read that Joe felt a little weak after the treatment, but this was not thought by the team to be particularly relevant.

It is not just in spasticity management where the clinical measurements may be misleading. Is a limited passive range of motion, as might be recorded on the plinth, a product of one muscle-tendinous unit or of multiple, is it due to the shortness of the musculotendinous unit or to its stiffness, is the muscular or tendinous part of the musculotendinous unit responsible? Currently, our clinical measurements are not only ambiguous but may reinforce a model of the underlying pathology that may not be accurate or relevant to the treatment of the individual. To improve the specificity of our assessments, our measurements must be aligned to a well-developed understanding of the presenting issues, whether it is abnormal activation or muscle deformity. Practically, that could mean introducing more technology into the clinical setting. For example, a combination of dynamic electromyography and dynamometry may be useful in assessing the contribution of the increased reflex sensitivity to muscle activation and resistance to stretch in passive and active conditions. Imaging could be used to estimate muscle length and volume, as well as stiffness and composition.

In the section on RCTs, we introduced the concept of the MCID, that is, the change in a variable that can be considered *clinically* significant. Such a statistic is as least as valuable in the clinic as it is in a research paper. There is a related measure called the minimal detectable difference (MDD), which is the change in a variable that can be considered *statistically* significant. MDD is calculated from the results of a test–retest study in the patient group of interest, while MCID may be determined directly from patient reports or from the opinion of a consensus panel or by regression with a variable considered to be important to the patient. There are few reports of MDD or MCID in the literature for the GMFM but these suggest an MCID of 1.7 points (Oeffinger et al. 2008) and an MDD of 2 to 3 points (Ko and Kim 2013). Andrew Sellers implemented the GMFM in evaluating Joe's response to Zenetec and found an increase of 2 points, 12 weeks after intervention. Andrew Sellers is a lovely chap and a caring paediatric physiotherapist, but should he have been so happy about the result? There are a couple of elements of Joe's story that should concern us. Although an assessment was performed prior to treatment, it was the first time that Joe had done a GMFM assessment, and the first time he had met Andrew. The GMFM is a capacity measure which requires the patient to give their best during the assessment. It is possible that the circumstances surrounding the first assessment may have led to an underestimate of the GMFM on that occasion leading to an apparent improvement at the second appointment. Andrew suggested to Joe that he expected the intervention to have a positive effect. Perhaps this encouraged Joe to make a greater effort the second time round. Perhaps Andrew scored Joe higher than he should have because of his desire for the treatment to work. To reduce this sort of bias, one might perform a second baseline (pre-treatment) assessment. Alternatively, the GMFM (and other outcome measures) could be a part of the routine practice at the clinic. In that case, any change in the GMFM may have carried a greater significance. Even with these potential non-clinical influences, the change in GMFM was barely clinically or statistically significant, which means that Andrew's enthusiasm for the 'result' may provoke further, possibly unnecessary, injections of Zenetec into Joe's musculature.

SUMMARY AND RECOMMENDATIONS

In this chapter, we have discussed the journey of a treatment from its testing in the research unit to its implementation and evaluation in the clinic. We have highlighted the difficulties in performing research, developing guidelines, and maintaining clinical practices that are transparent and free from biases.

Studies of treatments in cerebral palsy tend to show small mean effects and large variations in response. One of the problems for the clinical reader of RCTs and systematic reviews is the translation of the statistics presented on groups of individuals to the patient presenting in the clinic. The first step in improving this transfer of knowledge is to require researchers to generate numbers that have more clinical meaning than p-values and confidence intervals. It is possible for most reports to include probabilities of success or failure of the treatment and, in that way, enable the clinician and patient to have a more informed discussion about the risks and benefits of an intervention. The use of large multicentre databases of patient responses to existing treatments may further refine our decision-making by enabling us to calculate the likelihood of a positive or negative response to intervention according to the characteristics of the individual patient. Databases with several outcome variables spanning the ICF may help us to overcome a specific problem we have with prospective studies, that is, the lack of long-term outcome data. One barrier to successful implementation of big data approaches or to prospective studies is the selection of the dependent variables. We need a greater number of basic science studies to increase our understanding of the original injury and of the associated neurological and musculoskeletal maldevelopment (see Chapters 3 and 4). One purpose of these studies would be to create practical measures that could be used in research, and in the clinic, that were aligned with a more comprehensive model of the underlying pathology.

The clinician charged with the management of those with long-term musculoskeletal problems is interested in the stability or progression of the individual's condition and of their prognosis. Information that is sufficiently accurate and reliable is necessary to monitor progress, and to evaluate the success of intervention. In treatments that are continued or repeated, there should be an emphasis on determining whether the outcome variables have changed by a clinically significant amount, and that the patients themselves feel happy with their care.

The Musculoskeletal System
Not Just a Structure but a Process

The 'skeleton', as we see it in a museum, is a poor and even a misleading picture of mechanical efficiency. From the engineer's point of view, it is a diagram showing all the compression-lines, but by no means all of the tension-lines of the construction; it shews all the struts, but few of the ties, and perhaps we might even say none of the principal ones; it falls all to pieces unless we clamp it together, as best we can, in a more or less clumsy and immobilised way. But in life, that fabric of struts is surrounded and interwoven with a complicated system of ties: ligament and membrane, muscle and tendon, run between bone and bone; and the beauty and strength of the mechanical construction lie not in one part or in another, but in the complete fabric which all the parts, soft and hard, rigid and flexible, tension-bearing and pressure-bearing, make up together.

(D'Arcy Thompson, *On Growth and Form*, 1917)

WHAT IS A SYSTEM?

What do we mean when we talk about the musculoskeletal 'system'? A system can be defined as a group of elements which have a collective function, and which achieve this function through interaction. If we view the body as consisting of separate anatomical structures, it can be difficult to consider how altered development of one structure, the central nervous system, can influence the development of another structure, namely the musculoskeletal system. The key is to consider the body not as a structure but as a process; the systems involved are interdependent, and the interactions between the systems influence their development and output.

This chapter looks at the components of the musculoskeletal system, at how each component works, and at how the individual components interact to produce movement. We will see how these interactions mean that the musculoskeletal system is a process as much as a structure. In the next chapter, we will then look at how the musculoskeletal system develops from conception. Musculoskeletal function and development in the typically developing child is discussed initially, and we then consider how alterations in musculoskeletal development may occur in the child with cerebral palsy and may result in the clinical features we see. Although our understanding of the processes involved in typical musculoskeletal development is limited, it is still far greater than our understanding of the processes involved in the development of the musculoskeletal system of a child with cerebral palsy; discussion of the latter will as a result be more speculative than discussion of the former. Viewing musculoskeletal system development as an interactive process does, however, help us to suggest and identify possible mechanisms and interactions which may benefit from closer investigation and discussion.

LINEAR AND NONLINEAR SYSTEMS

We can start by looking at types of systems. If I put a litre of fuel in my car and am able to drive for a certain distance, then I can assume that if I put two litres of fuel in my car I can drive twice as far. This would be termed a linear system, where there is a direct or proportionate relationship between input and output. If, however, while driving my car, I listen to a piece of music which I enjoy, this does not mean that if I listen to another piece of music at the same time which I also enjoy that I will enjoy the combined music twice as much. The sound from both pieces of music will interact, with either positive interaction (synergy) or negative interaction (interference). In this case, the change in the output of the system will not be proportional to the change in the inputs. This type of system is termed a nonlinear system.

Most biological systems are nonlinear systems made up of a number of elements, which may in turn be systems in themselves. Biological systems are complex, show a degree of self-organisation, and have an ability to adapt to change in the environment through interaction between the components of the system. Because of this, an understanding of the individual elements or systems does not predict the behaviour of the overall system. The interaction between the parts of the system will result in what is termed an emergent property, which is not contained in the individual systems, and which may not have been predictable from knowledge of the individual components of the system. This sounds complex but is something we are familiar with in practice. Detailed knowledge of the properties of oxygen and hydrogen as gases, for example, and an understanding of how they may combine to form a molecule of water, would not predict the properties of water including wetness and surface tension, and would not predict how water would react to different temperatures to form either ice or steam.

Because of the nonlinear nature of a biological system, changing an element of the system may have a negligible effect on the function of the overall system or may greatly alter it; as the system is effectively more than the sum of its parts, it cannot be assumed that the effect of a change in one aspect of the system can be predicted. The interaction between the elements of the system and between the system and its environment also means that it may not be correct to say that one aspect of the system is controlling or directing the output of the system.

An example of an emergent property of a system, in this case the musculoskeletal system, is movement. Another example of an emergent property of a system, in this case an orchestra, is music. Looking at how musicians and their instruments interact to make music can help us to consider how to look at the musculoskeletal system. Let us look first at a single instrument, the cello, before moving on to look at the orchestra.

CELLOS AND MUSCLES

The cello, or violoncello as it was originally known, has a specific structure which has evolved to allow a specific sound to be formed and expressed. Different types of wood are used in the construction of a cello, such as an ebony fingerboard, a spruce top, and sides and a neck made of maple, because of the qualities of these woods in terms of strength and resonance. Cut-outs in the side of the cello make it easy to recognise but were developed to allow the bow to be used at greater angles by the musician. Even the decorative border of the cello, or purfling, has a function: it was designed to reduce the risk of cracks in the carved wood. These structural features taken together contribute to the sound produced by the cello, and will be well known to the cello maker or luthier. The sound of the cello, although easily recognisable, would not be something that would be predicted from analysis of the individual components in isolation but arises instead, or emerges, from the interactions between the components of the cello and the musician. Variation in the structure and components used will influence the sound produced. The musician will appreciate the structural features of the cello but may not be as concerned as the luthier with the precise details of the cello structure, and may instead be interested particularly in the interaction of these components and in the sound the cello makes. The type of bow used, and the way in which the bow is used by the musician, will also result in variations in the sound produced; all of the sounds will be recognisable, however, as coming from a cello.

As with the cello, each component of the musculoskeletal system has evolved to play a particular role within particular constraints; movement does not occur in a neutral setting but instead is influenced by gravity acting within and upon physical systems. The shape of bones and the structure of muscles are not random or arbitrary, they have developed in a way that allows us to produce movement in a given environment. The physical structure of muscles and bones influences the movement which is produced in response to activation of muscles by nerves. When the musician plays the cello, the note produced does not depend purely on the movement of the bow but instead on a combination of factors including the string involved, the position of the fingers, the structure of the cello, and the acoustic properties of the local environment. In the same way, the central nervous system does not have to specify the precise mechanics of a movement as these will be determined by the anatomy and structure of the body part which is moving, by the position of the other body parts, and by the external environment in which the person is moving. An astronaut giving the same motor commands to their lower limbs when on the moon, for example, would produce a different pattern of motion in comparison to the motion which would be produced on Earth.

The musculoskeletal system is frequently considered as a collection of separate tissues which act in a sequential causal pathway, which in turn ends in the production of movement. This is how some anatomy textbooks, for example, are compiled: there is a chapter on bones, a chapter on muscles, and a chapter on nerves. Each of these chapters may be detailed and informative, and the information is correct, but just as a physical description of the structure of a cello would not give the reader an awareness or perception of the capacity for the cello to produce music, a detailed description of the structure of the individual components of the musculoskeletal system may not help us to understand or appreciate movement. This approach does not diminish the importance of structure but instead looks at the musculoskeletal system from a different perspective; we want to look at the musculoskeletal system and movement from the perspective of the musician rather than the luthier.

Systems can work and interact at different levels and may be composed themselves of systems. The way in which the cello is played by the cellist, for example, can be seen as representing another level of interaction. Around 300 years ago, Johann Sebastian Bach composed a series of six suites for solo cello, which are perhaps the most well-known pieces for the instrument. Each suite consists of six movements, with a prelude followed by a number of dance movements. The suites are very popular, and there are numerous recordings available. The manuscript score for each suite specifies the relative duration of each note played but not the speed at which each suite should be played, leading to a wide variation in the speed at which the suites are played in recordings made by different musicians. There is no surviving copy of Bach's original manuscript but rather a number of secondary sources; the choice of manuscript and the resulting interpretation of the manuscript, including the speed at which each suite is played, will be influenced by the training, experience, and personality of the musician. We could consider the music played as emerging from a number of interactions: the components of the cello, the bow used, the individual playing style of the musician, and the interpretation by the musician of the manuscript score for the music. The music played by the musician in turn does not exist in isolation but will be influenced by the setting in which the music is played, the music played in this setting in turn may be interpreted differently by different listeners.

Individual musicians, each playing a musical instrument, can interact together in a group such as an orchestra; in this case the overall sound produced, as discussed further below, will emerge from the interactions of the musicians and the environment. In the same way, movement arises from the interactions between the musculoskeletal system and the physical environment, but even within the constraints imposed by gravity and structure a wide variation in movement is possible. Each musician in the orchestra, for example, will use the same underlying musculoskeletal system to produce different movements depending on the instrument each musician is playing.

The musculoskeletal system can be considered as an integrated system which produces movement, with the individual components of the musculoskeletal system functioning together much as musicians and their instruments in an orchestra produce music. From a systems viewpoint we can look at movement at a number of different levels; we can move from the molecular actions that combine to produce movement to how this motion interacts with our world to provide function.

THE ORCHESTRA AS AN EXAMPLE OF A SYSTEM

If we observe an orchestra playing music, our first impression may be that the music is produced from the orchestra through the gestures of the conductor. Each conductor will bring a certain interpretation or concept to the music but has to work with a range of factors including the physical nature of the instruments, the expertise and interpretation of the musicians, the interaction between individual musicians, and the physical setting of the performance. To the audience, the conductor may appear to be directly producing the music through their control of the orchestra, but it may be more accurate to say that the conductor is concerned particularly with the timing and overall expression of the piece of music, and provides suggestions or guides to the musicians about how the score should be interpreted rather than direct individual instruction. The implementation of these suggestions will be influenced, among other things, by the physical nature of the instruments; the same gesture of the conductor will produce a very different sound from the woodwind section and the string section. Even within a particular section of the orchestra such as the woodwind section, the sound produced in response to the gestures of the conductor will differ between instruments such as the clarinet and oboe because of their specific physical characteristics. We will see subsequently how the same input in the musculoskeletal system, namely innervation of the motor endplate in a skeletal muscle by an alpha motor neuron, will produce a different outcome depending on the architecture of the muscle which is activated, the site of insertion of the muscle, the position of the limb, and the environment in which the movement is produced. The same piece played by another orchestra, even with the same conductor, may sound different: the interpretation of the score by the musicians may differ and the interaction between the musicians may differ. The acoustic characteristics of the particular space or venue in which the music is played will also influence the sound heard by the listener. In the same way, although all of our musculoskeletal systems involve similar components and processes interacting in a similar environment, the movement produced by each musculoskeletal system is unique to that system.

If we consider the orchestra as a complex system, we can see that each component of the system is in itself a system with its own internal and external interactions. If, for instance, we consider the cello again we can see that the shape of the cello, the type of wood used in its construction, and even the varnish used will contribute to the sound produced by the cello, but it is the interaction of these components that is important in determining the sound the cello makes. These interactions in turn will be influenced by how the cello is played by the musician: the type of bow used, the direction of movement of the bow, and the degree of energy imparted to the strings will all contribute to the sound produced. The sound produced by the cellist will also be influenced by the music score, by the directions of the conductor, and by interaction with and feedback from the other musicians in that section. Each section, such as the string section, will interact with other sections of the orchestra. An experienced orchestra will learn a new piece of music through attention to the score but also through interaction between individual musicians under the overall guidance of the conductor. Awareness and feedback among the musicians are essential. Each musician must be aware at any point in time not only of the current note being played but also of the preceding note and the next note; they must also be aware of the overall expression of the music score by the orchestra.

CONSIDERING THE HUMAN MUSCULOSKELETAL SYSTEM AS A PROCESS RATHER THAN A STRUCTURE

Now imagine an orchestra where the musical instruments are not constructed and played but instead grow, develop, and make music by themselves, with each instrument developing its skill and ability to interact with the others as it develops, and with the resulting orchestra acting as a complex system which can continue to organise and develop itself while creating music through interaction with the environment in which the music is played and through feedback from the audience. This is what happens with the developing musculoskeletal system and movement. Such an orchestra or system does not need a single controller; in the words of Noble, there is no privileged level of causation (Noble 2012).

It may seem confusing and overly complex to discuss the musculoskeletal system in this way rather than simply provide a detailed list of the relevant components of the musculo-skeletal system along with an account of their structure. This would, however, be a little like describing the music heard at a concert by listing all of the musical instruments involved along with the physical structure of each instrument. In structural terms, a cello is an ordered but silent collection of wood and strings, and the Bach cello suites are simply symbols on paper. When a musician interacts with the instrument, we have music. When the component systems of the musculoskeletal system interact, we have movement. We can think of move-ment as music on a vast scale, as the outcome of a process involving the interaction of millions of molecules in a way that works within the constraints imposed at molecular, cellular, organ, tissue, and body system levels to allow us to perceive, interact with, and change the world in which we live. A child interacts with the world through their musculoskeletal system; muscles are involved in speech, hearing, seeing, eating, and touching, and help a child to play and interact with other children and with adults. Movement is an expression of who we are, and having an understanding or model of how movement happens and how it develops can be helpful in understanding how this process can change and how we can influence this change. Appreciating movement as emerging from interactions within a system and as not being isolated but instead occurring within a wider context, as with the musicians playing to the audience in a concert hall, allows us to move from the cellular level to the community in which the child is living and the world which they experience through movement.

ENTROPY, INFORMATION, AND THE CELL

If we are to look more closely at the musculoskeletal system and movement, the easiest approach may be to start with discussion of the cells involved. We are used to seeing illustra-tions of cells in which they appear as static and somewhat boring structures. The cell is the basic biological functional unit, and rather than primarily a structural component of a tissue, a cell is instead a complex system in which the interactions within the cell define its structure and function. These interactions together with interactions between similar cells give rise to nerves, muscles, and bones. To look at these interactions, we will first need to consider the concepts of information and entropy. Each of these concepts came from separate scientific fields: entropy from thermodynamics, and information from communications theory. More recently, they have been combined to look at information processing in biological systems.

The term 'entropy' was introduced by the German physicist Rudolph Clausius in 1865 and developed from the work of the French engineer Sadi Carnot who in 1824 showed that the efficiency of conversion of energy to work in a steam engine has an upper limit. In 1854, Clausius formulated what would later become the second law of thermodynamics: 'Heat can never pass from a colder to a warmer body without some other change, connected therewith, occurring at the same time' (see Smil 2017). The second law of thermodynamics states that the total entropy of an isolated system can never decrease over time, and that isolated systems spontaneously evolve towards thermodynamic equilibrium, the state with maximum entropy. This statement may seem obscure and may seem related to chemistry rather than to a biological system, but we will see that it has a particular relevance in a biological system. Entropy can be considered in this context as the degree of disorder within a system; a system where everything is equally disordered would be described as having high entropy, while a highly ordered system would be described as having low entropy. The second law of thermodynamics states that isolated systems evolve in a particular direction, from low to high entropy, and not in reverse. Consider a glass falling onto the floor: we can easily imagine the glass breaking into a large number of pieces. We would consider it highly unlikely that these pieces would spontaneously come together to reform the glass. In this situation, the intact glass could be considered as having low entropy while the fragments of the glass have higher entropy. When we think about it, this is a concept with which we are familiar although we may not have formalised it. We accept that a cup of hot coffee placed in a room will gradually cool, but see it as is unlikely that a cold cup of coffee will spontaneously warm up. We can accept that we could sit on a beach all our lives and watch the sand but are unlikely to see the sand spontaneously forming a sandcastle. So how is this relevant to discussion of the musculoskeletal system?

A living organism is a focus of low entropy in a higher entropy universe. Growth and development of the organism involve higher levels of organisation, which involve a reduction in entropy in comparison to the surroundings, which initially would seem to contradict the second law. The second law of thermodynamics applies, however, to an isolated or closed system where no energy can enter or leave the system. Living systems are open in that they can take in and release energy. The reduction in entropy in a living system requires the input of energy in the same way that building a sandcastle on a beach would require energy. As we will see in the next section, living organisms rely on low entropy energy, predominantly from photons in sunlight, for energy to maintain order within their systems. The capture of low-entropy energy, and the subsequent reduction in entropy within the organism, is accompanied by the release by the organism of high entropy energy as heat, which increases the entropy of the organism's surroundings. The reduction in entropy within a biological system is thus associated with a net increase in the overall entropy of the system of which the organism is a part, namely the universe. This means that each of us, as a biological island of low entropy, is contributing to the eventual end of the universe when entropy is uniformly high, and the lack of any low-entropy sources means that no further flow of energy or change is possible. At least, however, we can console ourselves with the thought that we are not breaking the second law of thermodynamics!

Entropy can be a confusing concept as there are a number of different approaches and definitions of entropy. In the late 19th century, Boltzmann and Gibbs used entropy essentially as a way of defining (in different ways) how much we did not know about a system such as a collection of gas particles in a closed space. If a system had very few possible configurations, and these were known, the system would have low entropy. A system where the molecules were randomly distributed would have high entropy. Another definition of entropy was developed by the engineer Claude Shannon in 1948 in the context of information theory regarding communications (in this case telephone communications) (Shannon 1948). Shannon looked at the information needed to describe a message and defined entropy as the amount of information contained in a message. A message consisting of a repeated single letter, such as AAAAAAAAAA, would not contain any additional information as the probability of each letter being A would be 100%, so the level of surprise on receiving each letter would be 0%. A message consisting of random letters would contain much more information and would need more information to be described. Shannon's concept of information also involved the context in which the signal was received; Cage's 4′33″, which we discussed at the beginning of Chapter 1, would have no Shannon information content (as it effectively consists of repeated units of silence) but resulted in considerable surprise in the audience. The Shannon concept of entropy, where low entropy corresponds to low information and increased unpredictability is related to increased information, can cause confusion when considered against the Boltzmann and Gibbs definition where high information is associated with low entropy, but each involves a different perspective. This can be appreciated by considering the different approaches to the definition of complexity (Deacon and Koutroufinis 2014). Shannon's work led to the independent development by Solomonoff, Kolmogorov, and Chaitin (reviewed in Deacon and Koutroufinis 2014) of the concept of algorithmic information content where the complexity or information content of a string of symbols is taken to be the length of the shortest algorithm or computer program that can generate this string. This is effective for communication but perhaps less so in biology as it would imply that putting a bacterium or skeletal muscle in a blender, so that all of the constituent molecules were randomly distributed, would make it more complex and would increase the information content of the mixture. This was addressed in part by Lloyd and Pagels, who developed the concept of 'thermodynamic depth', which described the evolution of a state rather than the state itself and was defined as 'the amount of information required to specify the trajectory that the system has followed to its present state' (Lloyd and Pagels 1988). While this concept will be very useful for us when considering an altered trajectory of development of the musculoskeletal system in children with cerebral palsy, it does not allow consideration of the different levels of organisation within a system which contribute to the overall complexity of a system. The concept of 'dynamical depth', which looks at such nested dynamical levels, has been developed by Deacon and Koutroufinis. These concepts are illustrated by Figure 3.1 where we can see that although

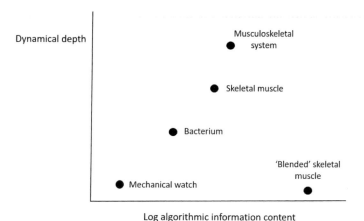

Figure 3.1   Dynamical depth and information content (see text for discussion). Adapted from Deacon and Koutroufinis (2014).

a 'blended' skeletal muscle will have more algorithmic information content, it will have much less dynamical depth than an intact skeletal muscle.

In general terms, the term 'information' when used in discussing systems is more likely to be used in the sense of the opposite of entropy meaning that an ordered system, where the distribution of the components of the system are known, will have high information and low entropy, while a highly disordered system will have low information and high entropy. Adami described information as a relative quantity which is always about something: 'what you don't know minus what remains given what you know' (Adami 2016). Information is thus a measure of the reduction in uncertainty following a measurement. This discussion may not seem relevant to living systems until we consider that organisms are complex systems which gather, process, store, and use information about their internal and external environments (Nurse 2008). A cell needs to identify and respond to local chemical, mechanical, and electrical stimuli; these could include nutrient substrate levels, hormones, ion currents, neurotransmitter levels, and mechanical stretch. Signalling pathways within the cell pass this information to cellular networks but also process this information in that the signalling molecules recognise the amplitude and duration of the incoming signal and produce a corresponding output signal (Azeloglu and Iyengar 2015). The processing and relay of the information depends on the organisation (or topology) of the network and on the interaction between the components of the network. Most of these pathways are part of wider pathways which interact with each other as part of a larger network. Components of the pathway are described as 'nodes', with interactions between the nodes described as 'edges'. In a biological system such as the yeast cell, information seems to flow particularly between what are termed 'key nodes', with a few key nodes forming a 'control kernel' in a network which influences the dynamics and hence the function of a network, moving it towards a stable end state known as an 'attractor' (Kim, Davies, and Walker 2015). This means that the flow of signals, or the information patterns, in a network is more important than the structure of the network. The flow of information in a network can be assessed using a concept known as 'transfer entropy' (Kim, Davies, and Walker 2015; Davies 2020). We could consider a node, which we could call node A, which can be either active or inactive. If knowing the pattern of activity and inactivity of node A helps us to predict what the next step will be, we can say that information has been stored in node A. If node A is connected to another node, node B, and if the current state of node A helps us to predict the state of node B, we can say that information has been passed from node A to node B.

As we saw above when we discussed entropy, building up information within a cell network, cell, or organism requires an input of energy as a system would otherwise tend towards a reduction in information and an increase in entropy. The creation of information or order was previously considered to be the step that required most energy, but it is increasingly recognised that the energy cost of information is related to the need to reset the system to its original state after every computation so that another cycle can be performed. Each cycle then acts as a 'ratchet', which allows accumulation of information (Boël et al. 2019). To consider this, we can consider that signalling molecules need to discriminate substrates in a noisy background, and in this way can be said to make measurements to gain information which is extracted from the environment. Each signalling molecule has a particular molecular configuration which shifts or changes to an alternative configuration on binding with a specific substrate. Before it can repeat the cycle, it needs to be reset to its original configuration; this is the step which involves energy. The main energy source within the cell, as we will see, is the high-energy phosphate bonds in adenosine triphosphate (ATP). The cellular network in this way exchanges the information gained for the entropy gained through the breakdown of the high-energy phosphate bond. In a similar manner, the formation of a molecule such as a protein in a cell involves an accumulation of information which is again driven by the conversion of low-entropy energy, the energy stored in the phosphate bond, to high entropy energy or heat. In this way, energy availability and consumption in a cell are not ends in themselves but instead facilitate information processing and flow within the cell for cellular processes. This is expressed well by Loewenstein (1998: xiv), who argued that Biological systems are information-processing systems and this must be an essential part of any theory we may construct' and by Brenner (1999: 1960–1965), who noted that 'information flow, not energy per se, is the prime mover of life – molecular information flowing in circles brings forth the organisation we call "organism" and maintains it against the ever-present disorganising pressures in the physics universe'.

Discussion of information processing and flow within a complex system can seem a little abstract and can be difficult to picture. We can return to the analogy of the orchestra. An orchestra is formed of individual components or 'nodes', made up of each musician and their instrument, which form interactions or 'edges' with other nodes. The layout of an orchestra, with the string section, woodwind section, and brass section, forms the structure or topology of the system, but the interactions between the musicians is what gives rise to music. A musical composition, such as a symphony by Beethoven, can be viewed as a non-equilibrium system where each note represents a state of the system; as the piece of music evolves, and as the notes change, each instrument can be said to transition between states with the simultaneous occupation of a set of states by all instruments creating the overall sound that we hear (Nicholson and Kim 2016). We can see music as an information flow, where within the context of Western classical music the succession of notes played by a particular instrument help us to predict the next note to be played and where the notes played by one instrument can help us predict the next note which will be played by another instrument. We can appreciate that an orchestra playing music will never be fully in equilibrium. Individual musicians, as discussed earlier, will respond to the other musicians in a nonlinear fashion with a continuous exchange of information; this interaction will move towards specific states of the system known as attractor states. We can define the output of the system, the music we hear, as a trajectory in a multi-dimensional space, whose axes or dimensions are defined by all of the variables which exert an influence over the system's current state and on its evolution in time (Schiavio, Maes, and van der Schyff 2021). This music, its trajectory over time, and the information contained will be defined by the interactions within the musicians within the orchestra, and will be driven by their energy input. Without this energy input, there would not be any sound; without the interaction between the musicians, however, there would not be any music.

Although analogies can be (and may have been) taken a little too far, we need to consider a cell in the same way that we consider an orchestra, namely as a system with a defined structure or topology whose function depends on interaction between these components. Discussion of cell function needs some discussion of cell structure, just as discussion of a piece of music is facilitated by an understanding of the musical instruments involved. In the next sections, we will look particularly at the cell membrane and at cellular proteins before going on to look at energy production and balance within the cell. For more information, the reader is encouraged to consult Harold for a detailed and very enjoyable review (Harold 2001).

THE CELL MEMBRANE: THE DIFFERENCE BETWEEN INSIDE AND OUTSIDE THE CELL

Cells are biological units enclosed by a membrane formed predominantly of two layers of phospholipid molecules. These are chains of around 20 carbon atoms with a phosphate group at one end of the chain; this makes the molecule both hydrophilic, meaning that it is attached to water, and lipophilic, meaning that it is attracted to other fats. The phospholipids line up essentially back-to-back so that the hydrophilic ends with the phosphate groups face the outside and inside of the cell while the fatty acid tails face each other. The presence of the cell membrane means that the inside of the cell can have a different environment to the outside of the cell, and this environment is sustained through control of passage of molecules through the cell membrane. This capacity to define a specific environment is crucial to cell growth and function.

PROTEINS: THE WORKHORSES OF THE CELL

The cell membrane and space within the cell contain proteins. Proteins are large molecules made up of smaller structures called amino acids. Each amino acid is joined to the next amino acid by means of a peptide bond, and the linear arrangement of the amino acids in a polypeptide is termed the primary structure of a protein. A protein also has a secondary structure because the different amino acids in the primary structure interact with each other and with the surrounding water molecules; this can result in the primary linear arrangement of amino acids forming a regular structure such as a helix. Further interactions between the amino acids, and between the protein molecule and water molecules, lead to further structural changes termed the tertiary and quaternary structure of the protein. The importance of the different levels of structure of a protein is that the cell does not need to contain all the information to guide the formation of the protein structure; instead, all that is needed is information to guide the formation of a linear sequence of amino acids, which will then interact and form a complex structure within a given cellular environment. This potential for structural development in a protein greatly reduces the amount of information needed to code for its structure; rather than specifying a complex three-dimensional structure, the cell need only code for a linear arrangement of amino acids.

The structure of a protein, as noted in the previous section, is due to the order or information which has been built into the protein when it was constructed. This information in turn allows a protein to 'recognise' a specific molecular substrate with a matching configuration. A protein with two stable configurations can shift from one configuration to another when it binds a substrate, acting in a way similar to a digital switch, which is either 'on' or 'off' (Loewenstein 1999). The vast number of proteins in the cell mean that there is a specific protein for each substrate molecule.

The ability of a protein to change its structure following an alteration in the structure of an individual amino acid, or in the secondary structure of the protein, may also allow it to act as a molecular motor. Kinesins, for example, are tiny molecular motors which transport other molecules and structures in the cell to where they are needed along self-assembling pathways made of structures called microtubules. Interaction between specialised structural proteins such as actin and myosin form the basis of muscle contraction through controlled movement at a particular site in the myosin molecule. This is discussed in more detail later in the chapter.

Some cellular proteins are integral to the cell membrane and act as specialised gates or filters to control the passage of charged molecules, or ions, through the cell membrane. Each ion carries a tiny electric charge so the passage of ions across a membrane is effectively an electric current. The cell membrane itself is not permeable to ions so by excluding (and actively pumping out) some ions a cell can develop and maintain a different concentration of ions across the cell membrane resulting in a gradient of electric charge or a voltage. Protein channels across the cell membrane can be activated by specific molecules which bind to receptor sites on the protein or in some cases may be activated by a change in voltage. A shift in the relative concentration of ions on both sides of the cell membrane can be brought about by selectively opening or closing protein channels; this effectively causes an electric current across the cell membrane, which can either cause changes in the activity of other proteins in the cell or can be propagated along the cell membrane as a signalling mechanism as we will see in both nerves and skeletal muscles.

Other proteins called enzymes facilitate chemical reactions in the cell and allow them to happen more quickly. Enzymes have a structure which allows them to bind the molecules involved in the reaction so that they can be brought close together to facilitate the resulting interaction. Enzymes greatly accelerate the synthesis and breakdown of complex molecules and allow the energy stored in molecular bonds to be captured and stored for use in cellular processes. As we saw earlier, after an enzyme facilitates a chemical reaction, it needs to be reset, or restored to its original configuration, by means of an input of energy. Enzymes can also act as 'switches', 'turning on', or 'turning off' cellular activities by means of either adding a phosphate group through enzymes called kinases or removing a phosphate group by enzymes called phosphatases. The high-energy bonds stored in ATP, which were mentioned earlier, and which are discussed in more detail below, thus allow this molecule to act as an energy currency within the cell.

Cellular proteins, by means of their three-dimensional structure and by interaction with other proteins, both provide a framework for the cell and allow the processes needed for cell life and growth. For this to happen we need two other essential processes: a means of making more proteins as needed, and a way to supply the energy needed for all of these processes.

HOW ARE PROTEINS FORMED IN THE CELL?

Complex organisms such as plants and animals are made up of what are termed eukaryotic cells. Each eukaryotic cell has a nucleus containing genes, which provide a template for the construction of the proteins needed for cell structure and activity. The nucleus has its own membrane, the nuclear membrane, which separates the nucleus from the rest of the cell but which has pores to allow communication and passage of molecules between the cytoplasm of the cell and the nucleus.

The genes in the nucleus are located within deoxyribonucleic acid (DNA). DNA is formed of structures called nucleotides, which contain a deoxyribose sugar, one of four nucleobases, and a phosphate group. The nucleobases consist of purine bases (adenine and cytosine) and pyrimidine bases (thymine and guanine). A sequence of three nucleotides is called a codon, and codes for one of the 20 most common amino acids. There are more possible combinations of codes than there are amino acids, so each amino acid has a number of different codons. A sequence of codons can code for the linear sequence of amino acids that makes up the primary structure of a protein, with other codons acting as indications as to where the sequence starts and ends. It is estimated that less than 2% of the human DNA molecule codes for proteins. The role of the rest of the DNA molecule is unclear; it has been termed 'junk DNA' but may contain control sequences such as those coding for molecules called microRNAs or miRNAs (discussed below), which influence how the proteins coded for by DNA are expressed and activated. In the cell, each DNA molecule binds to another DNA molecule in a double helix pattern: think of a ladder where the steps are formed of the bonds between the nucleobases (adenine binding to thymine, and guanine to cytosine) and the side rails are formed through the bonds between the adjacent nucleotides. The ladder is then twisted to form a helix.

We think of DNA generally in terms of chromosomes, which are paired structures with each chromosome consisting of a single DNA molecule. These molecules can be very long. To fit the DNA molecule, along with the other chromosomes, into the space available in the nucleus each double strand of DNA is coiled up around proteins called histones, and these chains of histones and DNA are then coiled again into a further compressed structure. The DNA molecules are wrapped and surrounded by protein molecules and ribonucleic acid (RNA) molecules to form a structure known as chromatin. In between times of cell division, DNA appears to have a dynamic structure in the nucleus in that each of the chromosomes appears to change its configuration depending on which genes are activated, with the relatively inactive part of the chromosome occupying the outer portion of the nucleus while the active portion of the chromosome is unwrapped and occupies the centre of the nucleus where different parts of the chromosome can interact with each other (Stevens et al. 2017)

The combinations of codons in DNA code for a linear sequence of amino acids which is formed in two major steps called transcription and translation. Transcription involves making a copy of DNA, and translation involves using this copy as a template to form a protein.

Transcription occurs through another nucleic acid, RNA. RNA is similar overall to DNA except that it has a different sugar (ribose instead of deoxyribose), and has uracil as a nucleobase instead of thymine. RNA occurs in a number of forms; messenger RNA (mRNA) is used to copy the codon sequence in DNA in the process of transcription, which happens in the nucleus. This involves the separation of part of the DNA double helix into its two component molecules through the use of an enzyme known as RNA polymerase. This enzyme makes an RNA molecule that complements the DNA molecule; this molecule of mRNA is then able to leave the nucleus through a nuclear pore and enter the cytoplasm where the process of translation occurs at a cellular complex called the ribosome. The ribosome binds mRNA and facilitates the binding of another RNA molecule known as transfer RNA or tRNA. The ribosome uses the mRNA as a template and fits the appropriate tRNA (and an attached amino acid) to the mRNA codons. Each time a tRNA is fitted to the mRNA template, its attached amino acid is brought close to the amino acid coded for by the previous codon, and the amino acids are joined to form a protein with a linear sequence of amino acids. The protein then develops a secondary, tertiary, and quaternary structure as discussed earlier.

BEING A CELL TAKES ENERGY

As we have seen, maintenance of the resting membrane potential and the synthesis of new cellular proteins through gene expression needs a continued and reliable source of energy. Most of the energy used by the cell is provided in the form of ATP. This molecule contains three high energy phosphate bonds. Enzymatic breakdown of ATP into inorganic phosphate and adenosine diphosphate (ADP; which can be broken down again into adenosine monophosphate [AMP]) provides energy for most cellular processes. ATP essentially functions as a unit of energy currency within the cell which is available to all processes as a ready source of energy. Once ATP has been broken down it is reconstituted by reforming the high-energy phosphate bonds so that they can be used again. This process involves harnessing the energy stored in electrons in complex molecules such as sugars, fats, and proteins, which are ingested by the organism and are delivered to the cell. In the case of glucose, part of this process can occur in the cytoplasm of the cell where it is termed glycolysis, but most happens in specialised structures in the cells known as mitochondria where it is termed respiration.

Glycolysis is the term given to the process in the cytoplasm in which a glucose molecule, which is composed of six carbon atoms, is broken down into two pyruvate molecules each with three carbon atoms. This provides enough energy to form four ATP molecules, but the reaction needs an investment of energy in order to occur. This is provided by the breakdown of two molecules of ATP for each glucose molecule, giving a net production of two ATP molecules per molecule of glucose. The pyruvate that is produced through glycolysis in the presence of oxygen is transported into the mitochondrion where two further processes occur, namely the citric acid cycle and oxidative phosphorylation. These processes together have the potential to provide a further 36 molecules of ATP from the two pyruvate molecules formed from a single glucose molecule, making cellular respiration more than 15 times more effective in producing ATP than glycolysis.

THE MITOCHONDRION: THE CELL'S POWER STATION

The mitochondrion provides most of the energy used by the cell for maintenance of cellular processes, movement, and growth. It has an outer membrane and an inner membrane, with an intramembranous space in between. The inner membrane forms folds or cristae which increase its surface area. Within the mitochondrion are enzymes which facilitate the capture of energy stored in the pyruvate. The first step is the further breakdown of pyruvate, a three-carbon molecule, to an acetyl group (containing two carbon atoms) through the removal of one of the carbon atoms. The acetyl group combines with coenzyme A (CoA) to form acetyl-Coenzyme A (acetyl-CoA). The acetyl group is then transferred from acetyl-CoA onto a four-carbon molecule, oxaloacetate, to form a six-carbon molecule, citrate. Citrate goes through a further eight steps involving 18 enzymes, during which two carbon atoms are removed, and oxaloacetate is formed again before another acetyl group is added by acetyl-CoA after which citrate is reformed and the cycle starts again. This cycle is known as the citric acid cycle or Krebs cycle and results in the formation of two ATP molecules for each glucose molecule (one ATP molecule for each pyruvate molecule). CoA also accepts acetyl groups from the breakdown of fats and amino acids and in this way allows these molecules to be used also to provide energy through the citric acid cycle.

As well as the direct formation of ATP as noted above, the citric acid cycle results in the capture of high-energy electrons each time a carbon atom and the associated high-energy bonds are broken. The high energy electrons which are released are captured through molecules such as nicotinamide adenine dinucleotide (NAD). NAD is positively charged (NAD$^+$) prior to accepting the electron (when it becomes NADH). The captured electron could be passed directly on to oxygen, which has a higher ability to attract or demand electrons, but a direct transfer would mean considerable loss of energy as heat. Instead, the captured high-energy electrons are passed onto and through complexes in the inner membrane of the mitochondrion known as the electron transfer chain, where the electrons gradually release their energy before they are accepted by an oxygen molecule. The energy captured from the electrons is used to move protons (hydrogen ions) across the inner membrane of the mitochondrion into the space between the inner and outer mitochondrial membranes. The resulting high concentration of protons forms a gradient which is released through an enzyme, ATP synthase, which forms new ATP molecules from ADP as the protons pass through before joining with the oxygen molecule to form water. Most of the ATP formed in the mitochondrion thus comes from ATP synthase through the action of the proton gradient, which is built up through capture of energy from electrons released from food.

This discussion focused particularly on energy flow as this is how these processes are generally considered. From our earlier discussion about information and entropy, however, this can seem confusing until we appreciate that the photons received from the sun have the capacity to support the build-up of information in the cell in the form of sugars as the photons have high information and low entropy. The range of wavelengths and photons within a photon from the sun are narrow, so it contains high information and low entropy. This type of energy has been termed 'free energy', meaning that it is free and has the capacity to do work. The information or order built up in glucose is in turn used in the cell to power the formation of another highly ordered molecule, ATP. Not all of the energy from the photon or from the covalent bonds in glucose is captured, the remainder is lost to the cell as heat. Heat is not 'free energy' as it is not able to do work; it consists of a range of different frequencies so has low information and high entropy.

There are other components to a cell which are termed 'organelles' including the smooth and rough endoplasmic reticulum (rough due to the presence of ribosomes) and the Golgi apparatus, which are involved in the processing of proteins formed by the cell for use in the cell and for export outside the cell, but the most important components of the cell for our purpose are arguably the cell membrane, the nucleus, and the mitochondria. The cell membrane provides a means of establishing and maintaining a specific environment within the cell by controlling the passage of molecules into and out of the cell and by providing a means by which external signalling molecules can effect change in cellular processes. The nucleus contains the chromosomes, which contain the templates for all of the proteins used in cellular activity. The mitochondria provide the energy in the form of ATP for most if not all cellular activity, and in this way provide the energy needed for growth; longitudinal

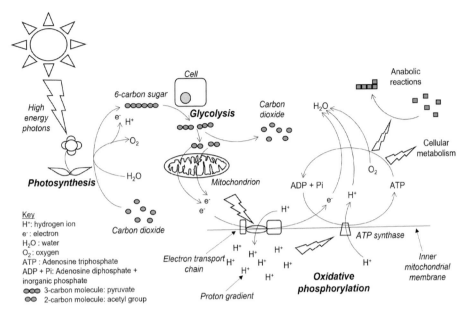

Figure 3.2   Energy flow in cells: using the sun to power cell growth and function. In photosynthesis in plants, the high information/low entropy energy from photons from the sun is used to form carbohydrates from carbon dioxide, using water as a source of electrons and hydrogen ions. In the cell, the six-carbon sugars (C6H12O6) formed through photosynthesis are broken down into three carbon sugars (pyruvate) during glycolysis; a further carbon atom is removed to form a two-carbon molecule which enters the citric acid cycle in the mitochondrion. This process is discussed in more detail in the text. High-energy electrons are captured during breakdown of the bonds in the sugar and are in turn passed through the electron transport chain before being accepted by oxygen: the energy captured from the electrons is used to create a gradient of hydrogen ions across the inner mitochondrial membrane. This gradient in turn powers an enzyme, adenosine triphosphate (ATP) synthase, which is used to form ATP which can then act as a source of energy within the cell. The carbon and oxygen atoms form carbon dioxide, and the hydrogen ions and electrons combine with oxygen to form water. The remaining energy is radiated as low-entropy heat (not shown).

growth velocity in children and adolescents, for example, is associated with skeletal muscle mitochondrial function (McCormack et al. 2011).

CELLULAR ENERGY BALANCE

We compared the cell to an orchestra in the previous section. A cell could also be compared to a city, with controlled transport and exchange of molecules between different parts of the cell, and with a structural framework which is constantly changing. In the same way that the interactions in a city are dependent on the economy and the availability of money, all of the activities within the cell (known as cell metabolism from the Greek term for change) are dependent on the energy balance in the cell, with ATP acting as a currency. Just as it would not be appropriate to start a large building project in a city if the city is low on funds, a cell needs to adapt its activity to the availability of energy substrates and the necessary components for protein synthesis. This close linkage is brought about by information flows between the mitochondria and nucleus through both signalling molecules and direct mechanisms.

In an energy rich environment, the availability of ATP in the cell increases, as does the concentration of citrate, the first stage in the citric acid cycle described above. The citrate formed is transported out of the mitochondrion and into the cytoplasm and nucleus through a shuttle system mediated by an enzyme called ATP citrate lyase and is converted in the nucleus by ATP citrate lyase back into oxaloacetate and an acetyl group, which again binds to CoA to form acetyl-CoA. The acetyl-CoA acetylates the chromatin in the nucleus, resulting in a change in chromatin configuration as noted above, which makes the DNA available for transcription. This in turn allows protein synthesis and facilitates cell growth (Wallace and Fan 2010; Gao, Díaz-Hirashi, and Verdeguer 2018). Conversely, when energy substrates are low, the chromatin keeps the DNA in a tightly coiled configuration so that it is not available for transcription, meaning that protein synthesis and cell growth are thus effectively blocked. Active deacetylation of histones and chromatin, which will block gene expression, is mediated through NAD^+, which was mentioned above as being part of the citric acid cycle, through a family of enzymes called the sirtuins (Gao, Díaz-Hirashi, and Verdeguer 2018). The NAD^+/NADH ratio, which will reflect the degree of ATP being produced in the mitochondrion, can in this way also influence cellular growth and gene expression. Lastly, gene expression can also be blocked through the binding of a methyl group (CH_3) to cytosine in DNA, termed DNA methylation. DNA methylation allows a stem cell, for instance, to suppress differentiation until it is needed. Most DNA methylation is stable but some is variable and is influenced by the energy balance within the cell (Gao, Díaz-Hirashi, and Verdeguer 2018).

SYSTEMIC ENERGY BALANCE

Each cell is influenced also by availability of energy within the system as a whole. The mechanisms involved in these intercellular information flows involve proteins which traverse the cell membrane and have binding sites for specific signalling molecules. When the receptor protein binds the signalling molecule it undergoes a change in configuration, which leads to activation of other proteins in the cell and to a resulting cascade which can influence cellular activity. An example is the hormone insulin; this is secreted into the circulation when carbohydrates are absorbed. It binds to the insulin receptor in the cell membrane and leads to a cascade beginning with the activation of an enzyme, tyrosine kinase, and leading to activation of two further enzymes, mitogen-activated protein kinase and phosphatidylinositol-3-kinase, which in turn affect gene expression and synthesis of molecules such as proteins, carbohydrates, or lipids within the cell resulting in cell growth. One of these pathways involves the mechanistic target of rapamycin (mTOR), which regulates cell growth and proliferation through two complexes: mTORC1 and mTORC2 (Laplante and Sabatini 2009). mTORC1 integrates signals from growth factors together with cellular energy levels, oxygen levels, and amino acids to promote anabolic activities within the cell including the synthesis of nucleotides for DNA transcription and the synthesis of lipids needed for cell membranes. mTORC1 also acts to increase mitochondrial function and numbers. mTORC2 acts within the pathway stimulated by insulin to promote cell proliferation and growth.

In the opposite situation where there is a lack of nutrients resulting in a reduced level of ATP within the cell, the reduction in ATP and the resulting increase in AMP leads to the activation of AMP-activated protein kinase (AMPK), which stimulates and promotes processes that produce energy, including the uptake of glucose and the breakdown of stored fats, while reducing processes that cost energy including protein synthesis and cell growth. The AMPK pathway involves the hypothalamus, liver, body fat, and skeletal muscle to help control energy balance over the whole body. This allows the cells in all of these organs to act as an integrated system able to respond flexibly to changes in level of activity or availability of substrates for metabolism. mTOR and AMPK in this way can be seen to represent opposing control systems which allow the cells in the body to respond flexibly to the availability of energy substrates. We will see later in the chapter that organs in the body such as muscle, bone, and fat interact with the liver and pancreas to allow a coordinated response to body energy levels.

A CELL IS A PROCESS AS WELL AS A STRUCTURE

The cell can thus be seen as a system or process which is not static but is instead dynamic. We have seen how the availability of DNA for transcription and gene expression is influenced by cellular energy levels and internal and external information provided by signalling molecules. Mitochondria are not fixed structures but instead multiply, combine, and divide depending on energy needs within the cell, a process known as mitochondrial biogenesis, and have the capacity to use the cell cytoskeleton as a framework to move to the sites in the cell where energy is needed. The cell membrane is also not static. Apart from the activity of the transmembrane proteins acting as ion channels and signal transducers, the membrane can expand to include a vesicle produced within the cell and in this way allow the export of proteins produced within the cell, as happens when a nerve releases a neurotransmitter, or can change shape to surround and engulf a bacterial cell as happens with phagocytosis.

The specialised processes happening in each cell in the body depend on the particular proteins produced through gene expression. Cells expressing similar or complementary genes are grouped through interaction into further complex structures or tissues which in turn combine to form organs and organ systems; in the musculoskeletal system these organ systems in turn interact to provide movement and function. To explain how this happens, we will look at the cellular processes in the main components of the musculoskeletal system, namely bones, muscles, and nerves, look at how the cells are grouped to form these components, and then look at how these components interact. We will see that the interaction and flexibility we can see in an individual cell extends through all levels of the musculoskeletal system and that, as with the cell, the musculoskeletal system should be viewed as a highly integrated process rather than a collection of structural components. It is useful to discuss individual aspects of the system but, just as discussion of the mitochondrion or nucleus in isolation will not adequately convey an understanding of cellular function, discussion of the skeleton, muscular system, or nervous system in isolation will not lead to an understanding of movement.

THE SKELETON: MORE THAN JUST A FRAMEWORK

We often consider bone as a static framework, almost inanimate in some ways, unlike muscle or nerve. The skeleton does provide a framework, with rigid sections upon which muscle can act to allow movement through joints. It is, however, very responsive to how it is loaded and has the capacity to remodel and to heal after injury. The skeleton is also increasingly viewed as an endocrine organ which senses and influences energy levels within the body. When discussing bone as a type of specialised tissue we use different terms including cortical bone and cancellous bone. Cortical bone is the name given to the tissue which forms the outer part of the bone and that takes most of the load imposed on the bone. The long bones of the limbs are essentially tubular and are formed from cortical bone in the midsection, which is termed the diaphysis. Towards the ends of the bone, where it widens out (the area known as the metaphysis) the central part of a bone is filled with small struts of bone called trabecula. This is termed cancellous bone. The trabecula are arranged and distributed in alignment with the pattern of loading of the bone.

Bone is a composite material made up of specialised cells in a mineralised connective tissue matrix of predominantly type I collagen, the main structural protein of the body, into which hydroxyapatite $(Ca_{10}(PO_4)_6(OH)_2)$ is laid down. The collagen fibres are formed by specialised cells called osteoblasts and are laid down in layers, with each layer ranging in thickness from 3 to 7 microns and with each layer aligned in a different direction to the underlying layer. This arrangement, termed lamellar bone, gives the bone greater strength. In developing bone, or when bone is formed initially in the process of fracture healing, the collagen fibres may be laid down without a specific alignment with the aim of providing a scaffold or framework to stabilise the bone and allow future remodelling. This is termed woven bone.

Each osteoblast forms bone around itself until it is enclosed by bone, after which it is termed a mature bone cell or osteocyte. Although apparently isolated in bone, each osteocyte is connected to other osteocytes in the bone by means of canaliculi through which long processes from each osteocyte extend and form connections with the cell membranes of the processes of other osteocytes through specialised connections called gap junctions. These connections extend through the bone and to the bone surface, where they communicate also with osteoblasts, and are thought to be involved in the response of the bone to loading and to the control of bone formation and resorption.

Bone which has been formed is constantly remodelled to match the demands on the bone. Remodelling of cancellous bone involves the removal of bone by multinucleated cells called osteoclasts, which secrete hydrogen ions which alter the local pH and allow breakdown and removal of the hydroxyapatite and the collagen. Osteoblasts then move into the resorbed area and deposit new bone. Remodelling also occurs in the dense and lamellar cortical bone. This is done by means of a 'cutting cone' of osteoclasts, which effectively tunnel through the bone, and which are followed by osteoblasts which surround themselves with lamellar bone and become osteocytes. Most of the tunnel is filled with bone apart from blood vessels in the centre; the arrangement of the lamellae give the structure a concentric appearance, which is termed the Haversian canal. The overall functional unit, with osteoclasts in front tunnelling the bone and then new bone being laid down by osteoblasts, is termed an osteon. Remodelling of bone allows the bone to respond to an alteration in loading pattern or to injury, but the cellular processes involved are expensive in terms of energy.

Bone also acts as a store of calcium and phosphate, and is closely involved in the control of systemic calcium and phosphate levels through interaction with the kidneys, gut, liver, and parathyroid glands. The space in the centre of bones contains bone marrow, which in turn contains stem cells which allow formation of red cells, white cells, and platelets. Although these functions of bone are very important, they are not discussed here.

Bones accept loads and act as rigid levers connected by joints through which muscle contraction can cause movement. The long bones of the limbs need to maintain a close balance between length and diameter. The ability of a structure to withstand bending under load is directly proportional to the diameter raised to the third power, and is inversely related to the length raised to the third power; this means that if a bone doubles in length it will also need to double in diameter to maintain the same resistance to bending (Rauch 2005). We also need to consider the shape of a bone in the overall context of its function. The femur, for example, has an anterior bow. In theory, when standing this results in an increased compressive load on the posterior aspect of the bone and an increased tensile load on the anterior surface of the bone than would be the case if the femur was straight and not bowed. The curvature in bone may, however, allow the bone to better withstand not just the loading imposed by body mass and gravity but also the loading imposed by the muscles working on and across the bone in response to the load imposed by body weight. It may also allow the bone to cope with a wide variation in the type and pattern of loading imposed (Milne 2016).

SKELETAL MUSCLE: THE PRIME MOVER

The skeleton is moved through the action of skeletal muscle. Skeletal muscle is also known as striated muscle because initial investigation of skeletal muscle by light microscopy showed a regular underlying pattern related to the distribution of the cellular proteins in muscle. Although the emphasis on muscle is often on the contractile component of muscle, muscle also contains specialised connective tissue extending through the muscle and connecting the contractile component of the muscle to a tendon, so that the shortening of the muscle which occurs through contraction results in movement of the part of the skeleton into which the tendon is inserted. We will look first at a muscle cell and then at muscle as a whole.

THE MYOCYTE: THE BASIC BIOLOGICAL UNIT OF SKELETAL MUSCLE

The skeletal muscle cell or myocyte is a specialised cell. It has the same cellular components which were discussed above, but these are ordered differently to a typical cell. A muscle cell or myocyte is very long (up to 40mm long in the human) with a diameter of 10 to 50 microns. The myocyte is a multinucleated cell with the nuclei found near the margin of the cell, just under the cell membrane which is termed the sarcolemma. The sarcolemma is also highly specialised; it contains areas which are called motor end plates, which are in close proximity to motor nerves, and it contains long deep invaginations into the cell, which are termed transverse or T-tubules. The T-tubules come into proximity with other specialised structures in the cell called the sarcoplasmic reticulum in which calcium is stored. The calcium concentration within a muscle cell is normally kept very low through active pumping of calcium into the sarcoplasmic reticulum.

The sarcolemma contains proteins which act as ion channels and allow the sarcolemma to maintain a negative charge or potential of -70 to $-90mV$ inside the cell with respect to the outside of the cell. The sarcolemma also contains ion-channels for sodium, a positively charged ion, which open when the voltage across the sarcolemma decreases, and which are thus termed voltage-gated channels. Outside of the sarcolemma are specialised structures called satellite cells, which contribute to muscle cell growth and can supply new nuclei to the cell. The mitochondria in a muscle cell are also ordered differently; there is growing evidence that the mitochondria are arranged in a continuous network which optimises availability of ATP throughout the muscle cell (Glancy et al. 2015).

The myocyte contains myofibrils which are made up of specialised structures called sarcomeres, which are arranged in series. A myofibril is around 1 micron in diameter. The space between the myofibrils is filled with T-tubules, sarcoplasmic reticulum, and mitochondria. The sarcomere is the site where muscle proteins forming thick and thin filaments interact to result in muscle contraction in what is known as the sliding filament theory of contraction. The sarcomere in mammals (including humans) has a resting length of just over 2 microns. It is bounded on each side by a structure known as the Z-disc, and has another structure called the M-line in the middle.

THE COMPONENTS OF MUSCLE CONTRACTION

Muscle contraction occurs through the interaction of a number of proteins, particularly actin, which forms the thin filaments, and myosin, which forms the thick filaments. The actin filament is composed of individual actin subunits, which link to form a long chain which is attached at one end to the Z-disc. The thin filament includes a structural protein called nebulin, which is entwined along the actin chain and is inserted along with actin into the Z-disc, and includes two more proteins called tropomyosin and troponin. Troponin is made up of three subunits, troponins I, C, and T. Troponin-C has a binding site for calcium and is attached to tropomyosin, which covers binding sites on actin for myosin.

Each myosin molecule is shaped like a golf club with a moveable head and a long tail. Myosin molecules are grouped around a very large molecule called titin, which extends through the thick filament from the M-line and is attached to the Z-disc. The portion of the titin molecule which runs between the end of the thick filament and the Z-disc is shaped like a coiled spring. The titin molecule is thought to help keep the myosin molecules organised and prevent overstretch of the sarcomere. Outside the sarcomere is another giant structural protein called obscurin, which surrounds the sarcomere at the level of the Z-disc and M-line and is thought to enhance sarcomere integrity. The sarcomeres are connected to the extracellular connective tissue by means of structures called costameres. These help transmit the force of contraction from the sarcomere to the external connective tissue, provide a site in the cell membrane for the attachment of receptors, and help maintain the integrity of the sarcolemma during muscle contraction.

Each muscle cell is enclosed in a layer of connective tissue known as the endomysium. Muscle cells are grouped into bundles or fascicles, surrounded by more connective tissue called perimysium, groups of fascicles are then surrounded by epimysium. Through

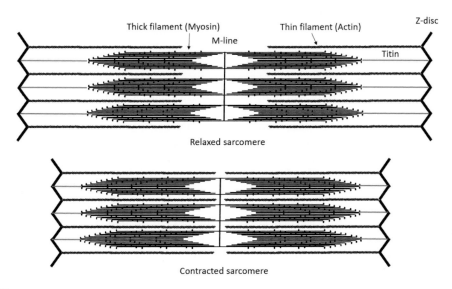

Figure 3.3   The contractile proteins of the sarcomere.

the costameres, endomysium, perimysium, and epimysium the force generated through muscle contraction in the sarcomere is transmitted through the muscle to the tendon and hence to the site of insertion of the tendon (Purslow 2002).

THE MOLECULAR BASIS OF MUSCLE CONTRACTION

Muscle contraction is initiated by acetylcholine, which is released by the motor nerve at the motor end plate (discussed in more detail below), and which travels across the space between the motor nerve ending and the sarcolemma, which is known as the synaptic cleft. The acetylcholine binds to a receptor in the sarcolemma leading to the opening of sodium channels in the sarcolemma. The concentration of sodium is higher outside the sarcolemma than it is inside, and the inside of the sarcolemma is negatively charged relative to the outside, so positively charged sodium ions flow into the cell along an electrochemical gradient. If enough acetylcholine is released and enough sodium ions flow in, the negative resting potential inside the muscle cell will decrease; if this happens, the voltage-gated ion channels mentioned above will open. This is a very rapid process involving positive feedback and results in the inside of the sarcolemma being briefly positively charged with respect to the outside. This depolarisation, or change in electrical charge, is termed an action potential. A muscle action potential lasts from 2 to 4 milliseconds after which part of the sarcolemma is refractory to further depolarisation for 1 to 3 milliseconds.

The action potential affects the voltage-gated ion channels in the sarcolemma resulting in a wave of depolarisation spreading along the sarcolemma very quickly (at around 5 metres/second). This wave of depolarisation is transmitted deep into the cell through the T-tubules where it is detected by a voltage-sensitive receptor, which activates a receptor in the sarcoplasmic reticulum leading to the release of calcium into the cell. The released calcium binds to troponin-C on the thin filament, leading to uncovering of the binding sites for myosin on the actin filament. This results in binding of the two myosin heads of each myosin molecule to the actin in what are termed cross-bridges.

The myosin heads have binding sites for actin and for ATP: the ATP which is bound is broken down into ADP and inorganic phosphate, and the energy released from the phosphate bond is used to change the configuration of the myosin head by around 5 nanometres. This is termed the 'cocked' position. When the binding site on actin is exposed by tropomyosin, the myosin head binds to the actin, releases the ADP and phosphate, and returns to its original configuration. This is termed the 'power stroke'. This movement or change in shape of the myosin head while bound to actin pulls the thin filament closer to the thick filament. Each myosin head then binds ATP, releases the actin, hydrolyses the ATP into ADP and phosphate, and is cocked for the next power stroke. Each sarcomere can shorten from a resting length of just over 2 microns (10^{-6} metres) to just over 1 micron, although the active range is generally a lot less, with the sarcomere length generally staying between 2 and 2.4 microns. The muscle contraction lasts while there is free calcium in the cell and ends when the calcium is pumped back into the sarcoplasmic reticulum.

MUSCLE ARCHITECTURE AND MUSCLE FUNCTION

The force that a sarcomere can generate is dependent on its length because of the interaction between the thick and thin filaments. A sarcomere can generate most force at its resting length as in this position the thick and thin fibres are optimally positioned to allow crossbridge formation. As the thin fibres are brought closer together, shortening the sarcomere, less force can be generated as the available binding sites for actin and myosin are already taken up. If a sarcomere is stretched beyond its resting length, the actin and myosin fibres are more separated and again there are less binding sites available. With increasing stretch, the passive tension in the sarcomere increases due to stretch on the sarcomeric proteins. The relationship between sarcomere length and force production has implications for muscle design as for optimal function each sarcomere needs to be at or near its resting length prior to muscle contraction. As the sarcomere structure is consistent throughout the muscle, changes in the force produced by muscles needs to involve either changes in overall muscle architecture, changes in the muscle proteins, or a combination of both factors.

Changes in muscle architecture affect muscle force output. Imagine one muscle formed of two fibres made up of eight sarcomeres each, and another made up of eight fibres each containing two sarcomeres. Would these miniature muscles work differently? In the muscle with shorter fibres the sarcomeres are working side by side (in parallel) so the force generated by each sarcomere will result in a greater force than that produced by the other muscle where the sarcomeres are arranged end to end (in series) but with a limited active range as each fibre is only two sarcomeres long. The other muscle, with the relatively longer fibres, would shorten more quickly because the speed of contracture of each sarcomere would add up, and the muscle would have greater active range. Overall, we can say that the speed of contraction of a muscle is related to the number of sarcomeres in series, and the force of contraction of a muscle is related to the number of sarcomeres in parallel. In most muscles, muscle fibres do not run in a linear fashion from one end of the muscle to the other but instead are inserted at an angle into the tendon known as the pennation angle. This means that muscle anatomical cross-sectional area is not usually an accurate way to assess the area of all the fibres in parallel so instead we use the concept of physiological cross-sectional area (PCSA), which is calculated by multiplying the muscle volume by the cosine of the pennation angle and dividing by the length of the muscle fibres.

If we take PCSA as an index of muscle force production and take muscle fibre length as an index of muscle range and speed of contraction, we can see some interesting patterns in the muscles of the human lower limb (Wickiewicz et al. 1983). The muscle with the largest PCSA, the soleus, has the shortest muscle fibre length, while the muscle with the longest muscle fibres, the semitendinosus, has almost the smallest PCSA. This is not surprising when we consider that the main function of the soleus is to move our body mass against gravity by plantarflexing the ankle, while the semitendinosus may work to rapidly flex the knee joint. Like each bone, each muscle has a unique architecture for a particular function. This reduces the demands of motor control as a similar pattern of activation of the soleus and semitendinosus will produce a different output in terms of force generation and in the resulting range and speed of movement. An analogy could be the different sounds produced by different musical instruments in an orchestra as discussed earlier following the same gesture by the conductor.

When considering muscle morphology, we also need to consider the tendon which, together with the connective tissue, is an integral part of the musculotendinous units. Tendons can vary in terms of length and diameter, and this affects their responsiveness to stretch. In a situation where precision of movement is a priority and where muscle contractions need to be transmitted accurately and directly, such as in the external muscles of the eye or in some of the small muscles of the hand, a short and relatively stiff tendon is effective. In larger muscles which are being loaded in excess of body weight, such as the gastrocnemius and soleus, a short stiff tendon would transmit the load directly to the muscle and could cause injury. In this case a longer tendon/aponeurosis complex can allow a more gradual delivery of the force, which in turn can protect the muscle fibres in return for a small reduction in the precision of movement. The ability of a muscle to set the level of tension in a long tendon may facilitate the storage and release of energy in the tendon.

Muscles cause rotation of joints. The effect of a muscle at a joint depends on how far the tendon is from the joint centre of rotation; to assess this, we use the concept of the moment arm of a muscle, which is the perpendicular distance from the line of action of the muscle to the joint centre. At the knee joint in humans, for example, the presence of the patella increases the effectiveness of the quadriceps muscle by moving the tendon a little further away from the centre of rotation of the knee joint. Because of the effect of the shape of the lower end of the femur on patellar position, a mild increase in knee flexion results in increased effectiveness of the knee extensor muscles. Similarly, a mild degree of flexion of the hip can increase the effectiveness of the hip extensor muscles. It must be remembered also that muscles have different actions depending on the position of the limb, and that muscles in the limb act together, so that the action of a muscle needs to be considered in the context of the activity of neighbouring muscles and in the context of the position of the limb and the trunk.

'SLOW' AND 'FAST' MUSCLES

The activity of a muscle may be influenced also by variation in the proteins in the muscle. Muscles can be graded according to the speed at which they contract and then relax after a contraction. One method used to classify human muscle is based on the predominant type of myosin heavy chain (MHC) isoform present; this method allows muscles to be considered as slow (predominantly MHCIβ) and fast (MHCIIa, MHCIIx) muscles, although in practice each muscle fibre may contain a range of different MHC isoforms. The MHC isoform expressed by a muscle cell is not fixed but instead varies depending on how the muscle is used; there is a shift towards a slower MHC isoform with more frequent and tonic muscle activation, whereas with reduced or phasic activity there is a shift towards a faster MHC isoform (Pette and Staron 2000; Schiaffino, Sandri, and Murgia 2007). A fast-twitch muscle will not just have a different myosin type but will also have differences in other proteins such as the calcium pumps used to return calcium to the sarcoplasmic reticulum after a contraction.

A 'slow-twitch' muscle fibre reaches peak force production slowly and relaxes slowly but can maintain force production for prolonged periods. A 'fast-twitch' muscle fibre produces force more rapidly and relaxes more rapidly but may not be able to sustain this force due to the increased energy demands involved. Energy is needed within the muscle cell for actin/myosin interaction, for rapid storage of calcium in the sarcoplasmic reticulum after contraction, and for repolarisation of the sarcolemma following the action potential. This energy is provided by ATP, although at the start of a muscle contraction creatine phosphate may be used as an energy source with the phosphate bond being reformed subsequently. Glycolysis, as discussed earlier in the chapter, happens almost immediately after muscle contraction while ATP generation from mitochondria takes longer to build up. This means that for very short and high levels of force generation there will be greater reliance on glycolysis from stored glycogen in the muscle. Baker et al. estimated that during a 30-second sprint, breakdown of creatine phosphate accounts for 23% of energy provision, glycolysis for 49%, and mitochondrial respiration for 28% of the energy provided (Baker, McCormick, and Robergs 2010). During a 10-second maximal sprint it has been estimated that 53% of the energy is provided from creatine phosphate, 44% from glycolysis, and only 3% from mitochondrial respiration.

SKELETAL MUSCLE IS DYNAMIC AND RESPONSIVE

Skeletal muscle is a highly adaptable tissue, and is able to respond to altered demand by changes in the number and type of proteins involved in muscle contraction, and in the number of mitochondria present, through expression of genes within the cell nucleus. Factors influencing muscle gene expression include the pattern of neuronal activation, the energy substrates available, and the presence of local hormones and growth factors. The mitochondrial content of the sarcomere, and the ability of the sarcomere to use energy substrates such as glucose or fat, appear to be influenced by pathways within the cell which are sensitive to the pattern of neuronal activation such as those involving the calcineurin-nuclear activated factor of T-cells system (Schiaffino, Sandri, and Murgia 2007) and calmodulin. These pathways are thought to be responsive to calcium levels within the cell; as we saw earlier, calcium release from the sarcoplasmic reticulum triggers muscle contraction and the frequency, duration, and level of the changes in calcium concentration within the cell may act as a marker for cell activity. The calcineurin-nuclear activated factor of T-cells pathway appears to be important in determining the type of MHC synthesised in the cell; this in turn influences the contraction speed of the muscle as noted above so that a muscle which is used frequently can shift its contractile protein expression to a slower phenotype and can alter its ATP production through an increase in mitochondria (Pette and Staron 2000; Schiaffino, Sandri, and Murgia 2007). Mitochondrial uptake of calcium during muscle contraction both appears to enhance mitochondrial function and, by activating a number of intracellular pathways, enables the mitochondria to directly influence gene expression by the muscle cell nuclei and in this way influence muscle growth and protein synthesis (Mammucari et al. 2015).

A muscle fibre may be viewed as a complex adaptive system influenced by a number of factors including innervation, the mechanical load imposed, and the presence of local or systemic growth factors. Of these factors, the most important appears to be the pattern of neuronal activation and the resulting ionic changes (particularly in calcium levels) and mechanical stresses associated with contraction. Neuromuscular electrical stimulation after chronic spinal cord injury in humans has been shown to lessen reduction in muscle volume and the reduction in muscle oxidative capacity (Biering-Sørensen et al. 2009). A focal impairment of muscle growth with replacement of the muscle fibres by fat and fibrous tissue was noted in neonatal mouse models of brachial plexus palsy following neurotomy (Nikolaou et al. 2011) or focal muscle denervation using botulinum toxin A (Kim et al. 2009). Denervation of the tibialis anterior in adult rats by using botulinum toxin resulted in significant changes in gene expression throughout the muscle including a reduction in mitochondrial biogenesis and increased fibrosis associated with muscle atrophy (Mukund et al. 2014), and resulted in reduction in the volume of contractile tissue in rat muscle, an increase in the volume of noncontractile tissue, and a loss of muscle structure (Pingel et al. 2017). These studies suggest that the intracellular molecular events which occur during muscle contraction, and which are blocked by denervation, play an important role in maintaining the integrity of the muscle cell and in facilitating its response to imposed demands.

Muscle denervation, limb immobilisation, systemic inflammation, and starvation result in active muscle protein degradation and muscle atrophy (Gundersen 2011). Cast immobilisation, for instance, will lead to a reduction in muscle fibre protein synthesis and a shift towards protein degradation within the muscle fibre. This is a process which involves tagging of muscle fibres by ubiquitin prior to proteolysis and in which myostatin, a local hormone or myokine produced by muscle, appears to be involved (Gundersen 2011). Cast immobilisation of the quadriceps in the human results in a reduction in protein synthesis within 48 hours (Urso et al. 2006) and also in a reduction of the normal protein synthesis response of muscle to ingested amino acids (Glover et al. 2008). Growth factors may have different actions on different components of the muscle; myostatin, which inhibits muscle fibre growth, is important in muscle repair and appears to promote growth of the connective tissue component of muscle (Zhu et al. 2007). Insulin-like growth factor 1 is released by the muscle when active and promotes protein synthesis within the myocyte through pathways involving mTOR (Clemmons 2009; Otto and Patel 2010).

Passive stretch may lead to a short-term alteration in the length of the noncontractile component of muscle but does not appear in isolation to promote growth or development of the contractile component of muscle. This is to be expected given the complexity of the interactions involved in muscle protein synthesis and the role of cellular and systemic energy levels as discussed above. Muscle protein synthesis is suppressed during periods of active contraction, but there appears to be a subsequent increase in protein synthesis (Atherton et al. 2009). Cultured muscle cells show a prolonged inhibition of protein synthesis after mechanical stretch without activation (Atherton et al. 2009). In the rat soleus repeated passive stretch appears to promote expression of the atrophy pathway (Gomes et al. 2006).

MUSCLE INNERVATION

Each skeletal muscle fibre is innervated by a single alpha motor neuron (αMN), with each αMN innervating a number of muscle fibres. The αMN and its associated muscle fibres are known as a motor unit (MU). There is a close relationship between the size of a MU, the size of the αMN, and the force produced by the MU. Small MUs generally have a small number of slow fibres innervated by a small αMN, and large MUs generally have a large number of fast fibres innervated by a large αMN. These differently sized MUs are distributed throughout the muscle in a manner that allows the graded development of the force of contraction of the muscle (Henneman and Olson 1965). When a muscle contracts, small MUs are initially activated. As the force required from the muscle increases, larger MUs are recruited and the rate of contraction of individual MUs is increased. This allows smaller muscle fibres with greater endurance to be used more frequently, and reserves the energy-expensive large MUs for movements where speed and force of contraction are important. The distribution of differently sized MUs throughout the muscle and the close integration between the contractile and noncontractile components of the muscle facilitate the smooth transmission of the force generated by the contractile component of muscle to the noncontractile component and hence to the muscle tendon and the tendon insertion.

CONTROL OF MOVEMENT: THE NERVOUS SYSTEM

We often consider the musculoskeletal system as consisting just of muscles and the skeleton, but controlled movement needs a combination of controlled activation of the muscles and a mechanism to collect and integrate feedback from the movement of the muscles and joints. Because of this, discussion of the musculoskeletal system without some discussion of the neural mechanisms involved would be incomplete. A detailed description of the composition and function of the central nervous system is outside the scope of this chapter, but some limited discussion may be helpful if we are to consider musculoskeletal function. We will start by looking at the nerve cell and then consider how the nervous system is built up.

THE NEURON: THE BASIC BIOLOGICAL UNIT OF THE NERVOUS SYSTEM

The nerve cell or neuron is a specialised cell with the same components we have previously discussed but with a specific structure which allows the integration and communication of signals to and from the central nervous system. Nerve cells can be considered as being composed of three types: sensory or afferent nerves, which carry information towards the central nervous system; motor or efferent nerves, which activate a muscle fibre or secretory gland; and interneurons, which connect with other neurons in the central nervous system.

Nerve cells vary in shape and pattern but generally have a body or soma which contains the nucleus, have an area through which signals enter the nerve (in a motor neuron this can be in the form of many thin branched processes called dendrites, while in a sensory neuron this may be a mechanoreceptor in the skin), and a single process called an axon through which electrical signals can be communicated to another nerve or to an effector organ such as a muscle through small endings known as synaptic boutons or terminal boutons. The nerve cell membrane, like the sarcolemma in the muscle cell, has proteins crossing it which act as ion pumps and channels, and has a difference in voltage with the interior of the cell being negatively charged (resting potential of around -70mV) with respect to the outside. The junctions between nerves are called synapses and the space between the synaptic bouton and the dendrite is called the synaptic cleft.

We saw earlier that initiation of muscle contraction through the generation of an action potential in the sarcolemma was essentially an 'all or nothing' process. Nerve cells work differently in that the cell integrates the inputs from other axons which are received on its dendrites. These inputs can work to move the resting potential further away from the threshold for commencement of an action potential (around -40mV) in which case they are termed inhibitory postsynaptic potentials (IPSPs), or the inputs can move the resting potential closer to the threshold potential in which case the inputs are called excitatory postsynaptic potentials (EPSPs). The alteration in the resting potential in each case is caused by the effect of a chemical called a neurotransmitter, which is released by the terminal bouton of the axon and travels across the synaptic cleft to act on a receptor in the dendrite.

The main inhibitory neurotransmitter in the brain is gamma aminobutyric acid and the main excitatory neurotransmitter is glutamate, although these neurotransmitters may have other actions depending on the type of neurons involved. An αMN in the spinal cord will typically have around 10 000 inputs, 8000 on the dendrites and 2000 on the cell body (Feher 2017). The effect of an IPSP or EPSP lasts for around 15 to 20 milliseconds, so repeated signals in the same area can have an additive effect, which is termed temporal summation, or may add to the effect of IPSPs or EPSPs in surrounding areas of the dendrite, which is termed spatial summation. The area of the cell body closest to the axon is known as the axon hillock; this has a higher concentration of sodium channels than occur in the dendrites and is relatively more sensitive to changes in resting potential caused by IPSPs or EPSPs. If enough EPSPs are received to lower the resting potential enough to allow an action potential, then an action potential will begin in the axon hillock and will be propagated along the axon.

THE BASIS OF NEURONAL SIGNALLING: THE ACTION POTENTIAL

The action potential in a neuron, as in the myocyte, involves the opening of voltage-gated sodium channels. This is a positive feedback mechanism, with more channels opening as the voltage drops further, and it leads to an almost explosive change in the resting membrane potential with the interior of the cell becoming positively charged with respect to the exterior. This is corrected by opening potassium channels through which positively charged potassium ions can flow out, after which a sodium/potassium pump restores the resting potential. By that time, the local current associated with the flood of sodium ions has triggered adjacent voltage-gated ion channels resulting in propagation of the action potential along the axon. The rate at which an action potential travels along an axon varies according to factors such as the axon diameter (less current leak from wider axons) and temperature but is estimated as being between 0.5 and 10 metres/second.

This speed of transmission is greatly increased and the energy cost of transmitting an action potential is greatly reduced by the presence of myelin. Myelin is a lipid-rich substance formed by cells in the central nervous system called oligodendrocytes and by cells in the peripheral nervous system called Schwann cells. These cells essentially wrap a number of layers of myelin around the axon; these effectively insulate the axon and prevent current leakage so that the local current changes induced by the action potential do not have to move steadily along the axon but instead can 'jump' between the parts of the axon which are not covered in myelin (the nodes of Ranvier). This type of conduction, called saltatory conduction, speeds the transmission of the action potential to 150 metres/second.

When the action potential reaches the end of the axon, it activates voltage-gated calcium channels in the nerve cell membrane. There is an influx of calcium into the nerve ending resulting in fusion of stored vesicles containing neurotransmitter with the cell membrane at the synapse, after which the neurotransmitter is released into the synaptic cleft. If the target is a muscle, muscle contraction may be initiated as we have seen earlier. If the target is the dendrite of another neuron, the neurotransmitter released will cause IPSPs or EPSPs and in this way influence the output of another neuron.

PROVIDING THE ENERGY FOR NEURONAL SIGNALLING

Almost all of the energy needs of the neuron, in terms of availability of ATP, are met by mitochondria. Mitochondria form in the nerve cell body and are then transported by antegrade transport along microtubules in the axon to the synaptic bouton, while older and less functional mitochondria are returned from the bouton and axon by retrograde transport for recycling. In the case of a neuron such as an αMN with a cell body 30 microns in diameter and an axon 1 micron in diameter and 1 metre long, Saxton and Hollenbeck (2012) compared the situation to standing in a lecture hall 30m in diameter with a 1m diameter pipeline extending to a terminal 1000km away through which new machinery and supplies needed at the terminal must be transported while older or used equipment must be returned for recycling.

Niescier et al. measured the speed of a mitochondrion undergoing antegrade transport in an axon as 0.5 microns/second, which would mean that it would take a mitochondrion almost a month to travel from the cell body in the ventral horn of the spinal cord to the motor end plate (Niescier et al. 2016). Any alteration in mitochondrial function at the level of the motor end plate in an αMN may thus take some time to be resolved or repaired by the cell body. Similarly, an increase in energy demands such as may be needed in longitudinal growth of the axon or in repair of injury may take more time for a longer axon than would be the case with a shorter axon. The presence of myelin on an axon reduces the energy cost of transmission within the axon, but the formation of myelin involves a large energy investment by the system because of the need to synthesise the proteins and lipids needed in the formation of myelin; it also involves energy consumption for the maintenance of the resting membrane potential in the oligodendrocytes. Because of this, the presence of myelin may greatly increase the speed of transmission of the action potential by the nerve but may not alter the energy needed in comparison to an unmyelinated nerve (Harris and Attwell 2012).

THE CONCEPT OF UPPER AND LOWER MOTOR NEURONS

The importance of the nervous system lies not so much with the individual neurons as with their connectivity. To aid in clinical assessment and diagnosis we often talk about the upper motor neuron (by which we usually mean the pyramidal cell in the motor area of the cortex and its long projection to the spinal cord) and the lower motor neuron (by which we mean the αMN). We have seen that rather being connected exclusively by a single neuron the αMN may have up to 10 000 synaptic inputs. This suggests that for many αMNs the corticospinal axon may essentially suggest a course of action but will join with input from other neurons in determining whether or not an action potential will be generated in the αMN.

In a similar manner, we often discuss and test for a monosynaptic reflex where a specific sensory input results in a rapid motor output, such as when the relaxed patellar tendon is suddenly stretched with a tendon hammer. In this situation, the stretch of the muscle is thought to be detected by specialised sensory organs within the muscle, namely muscle spindles and the Golgi tendon organ. The Golgi tendon organ is a sensory receptor at the junction between the muscle and tendon, which is activated by stretch. The muscle spindle consists of muscle fibres, a motor neuron, and a sensory neuron. This motor neuron, which is generally described as a gamma motor neuron, is smaller and has a reduced speed of nerve conduction in comparison to an αMN, and is thought to set the level of tension in different parts of the muscle spindle so that changes in muscle length and speed of contraction can be detected.

There are differing theories about how these organs work and whether they are active when a muscle is active or when it is at rest, with the muscle tendon reflex being attributed to both or either organ. A review of the literature did not show any consensus as to which of these sensory receptors was involved in the tendon reflex and whether the muscle fibres in the muscle spindle (called the intrafusal fibres) were active without concomitant activation of the alpha motor neurons.

THE CENTRAL NERVOUS SYSTEM REALLY IS A SYSTEM …

The upper and lower motor neuron model portrays the spinal cord as a sort of relay station where these neurons meet. In a similar manner, we often consider the spinal cord as simply a relay station for the transmission of sensory information to the brain. The spinal cord instead appears to be able to integrate sensory input and coordinate motor output through collections of interneurons that are suggested to form central pattern generators which facilitate movements such as walking. This has recently been reviewed by Arber and Costa who suggested that the central nervous system works as an integrated system, with the cortex 'broadcasting' the intention to move through the system, the choice of movement and commitment to move happening in the basal ganglia, the integration of motor commands and the selection of the appropriate spinal circuits happening in the brainstem, and resulting commands being sent to executive centres in the spinal cord through which the movement is executed (Arber and Costa 2018). Wolpert et al. suggest that this selected movement will then be monitored, and the predicted movement compared with the actual movement, with integration of sensory input and motor output occurring in the cerebellum (Wolpert, Diedrichsen, and Flanagan 2011).

... AND IS PART OF A LARGER SYSTEM WHICH INCLUDES THE SKELETON AND MUSCLES

Wolpert et al. discussed a number of potential sources of variability between a predicted and actual movement which could be considered in the context of an athlete involved in a sport such as football (Wolpert, Diedrichsen, and Flanagan 2011). The first potential source of variability is uncertainty; it may be difficult for us to predict exactly how the other player will kick the ball and where the ball will go. The second source of variability is redundancy; with around 600 muscles in the body, each of which we can either activate or not, we have 2^{600} choices about how we will activate them. The third source of variability is noise in terms of potential error in both the motor output and the sensory signal. The fourth source is the inherent delay in neural transmission; even moving along a myelinated axon at a maximum speed of 150 metres/second it will take time for a sensory input to be received and processed and for a motor response to be calculated and activated. An example would be a goalkeeper trying to save a penalty: by the time he has worked out the direction in which the ball is moving, it would already be behind him in the net so the goalkeeper's only option is to make a prediction of the trajectory of the ball based on the available information and on experience. Another source of uncertainty relates to possible changes in muscle function and motor response for instance due to fatigue. This is termed non-stationarity. Finally, the musculoskeletal system acts in a nonlinear fashion; the central nervous system can make a suggestion, but the resulting movement will depend not just on muscle activation but on the mechanics and inertial properties of the limb and the effect of gravity. Wolpert et al. suggest that we involve different circuits in the central nervous system, including the cerebellum, to both develop a plan of movement and also predict the sensory consequences of movement so that both can be compared in a process of ongoing motor learning. Viewed in this context, information from the muscle and tendon about the force and speed of contraction would be essential in the central control of movement.

INTERACTIONS WITHIN THE MUSCULOSKELETAL SYSTEM: BALANCING ENERGY AND GROWTH

In all of the components of the musculoskeletal system there is a common thread, namely the need to provide energy to allow the system to function and the need to balance growth with available energy reserves. We have seen in muscle cells that there is close integration between the mitochondria and the nucleus. We have also looked at the interaction between the mTOR pathway, which promotes further growth and development, and the AMPK pathway, which suppresses energy-expensive activities and increases the breakdown of cellular energy stores depending on the availability of energy substrates. These pathways are not specific to muscle cells. AMPK acts to improve the availability of energy to the body by increasing glucose uptake, lipid oxygenation, and mitochondrial biogenesis in muscle. It acts on the liver to decrease glucose production and lipid synthesis, while promoting lipid breakdown. It acts on the pancreas to reduce insulin secretion and circulating insulin levels, while reducing both breakdown and synthesis in adipose tissue (Long et al. 2007). It acts in the nervous system to reduce or stop myelination of axons. mTOR acts throughout the body to promote cell growth and proliferation, while acting on muscle, liver, and fat to increase energy storage.

There is increasing evidence that muscle, bone, and adipose tissue interact as endocrine organs. Leptin is a hormone released by fat; there are leptin receptors in the hypothalamus which influence bone mass through sympathetic output to bone (Corr, Smith, and Baldock 2017). Adipose tissue appears to secrete a number of hormones that are involved in glucose and lipid modulation, including adiponectin, which reduces osteoblast proliferation and bone formation (Kajimura et al. 2013). A contracting muscle releases a range of active agents, termed myokines, which have both local and systemic effects. They act locally on energy substrate oxidation, cell hypertrophy, angiogenesis, inflammatory processes, and regulation of the extracellular matrix. They act systemically on adipose tissue to increase breakdown and reduce cell mass, on the liver and on the pancreas to enhance glucose metabolism, on the immune system to improve function, and on bone to increase bone formation and mineralisation (Hoffmann and Weigert 2017). Bone has also been found to secrete two hormones. Osteocalcin is produced by osteoblasts and acts on the islet cells in the pancreas to increase insulin production and insulin secretion, acts on adipose tissue to increase adiponectin release, and acts on skeletal muscle to increase insulin sensitivity and glucose uptake. It also appears to act on the testes to increase testosterone production (Karsenty and Olson 2016).

These interactions may explain why some interventions may have an unexpected effect. In healthy young adult volunteers, 6 to 7 days of strict bed rest resulted in moderate deterioration in oral glucose tolerance and an increase in both fasting plasma insulin concentration and the insulin response to an oral glucose challenge by more than 40%. This appeared to occur primarily in skeletal muscle as no changes were noted in the action of insulin on the liver (Stuart et al. 1988). The use of a daytime knee splint for 7 days by five young adults was noted to reduce the effect of insulin on glucose uptake in the quadriceps muscle (Richter et al. 1989). A subsequent similar study (Abadi et al. 2009) in 24 adults showed reduction in muscle volume and muscle strength after 14 days of immobilisation, which was associated with a wide range of changes in gene expression, including downregulation in genes involved in mitochondrial function and protein synthesis, and upregulation of genes involved in protein degradation. These findings may be particularly relevant to children with cerebral palsy with altered muscle development and reduced voluntary movement.

CONSIDERING MUSCULOSKELETAL GROWTH AS A PROCESS

The concept of movement, or function, as a process involving interaction within and between systems allows us to view movement as an emergent property of this interaction. We can see this process as having a trajectory, where the current state of the process influences future states and is in turn dependent upon the previous state of the process. This seems obvious when we consider an activity such as movement but can also be applied to the systems which interact to form a movement such as muscles, bones, or nerves. We generally consider muscle or bones as fixed structures but can consider them also as processes or systems with a current state which is dependent on previous states of the system and which constrains future states of the system. We take this approach already implicitly when we consider musculoskeletal growth, when we appreciate that bones and muscles are not fixed structures but instead change in size with growth, and when we consider that the trajectory of this change can be influenced by external factors and by the current state of the process. Musculoskeletal development was compared earlier in the chapter to the development and interaction of instruments in an orchestra without the need for musicians or a conductor. If we consider the musculoskeletal system as a complex system then we also need to consider how it develops and need to consider how an alteration in development could explain some of the clinical findings in children with cerebral palsy. This is the focus of the next chapter.

Musculoskeletal System Development
Typical and Altered Trajectories

In the previous chapter, we looked at the musculoskeletal system as a set of interacting processes and systems giving rise to movement. In this chapter, we look at how such interaction can give rise to musculoskeletal growth and development, and how this development could be altered in a way that could result in the changes we see in the musculoskeletal system of children with cerebral palsy. Before doing this, it may be helpful to review some of the concepts involved and to consider sources of variation in developmental outcomes.

CONCEPTS IN CELL DEVELOPMENT: EPIGENETICS, STATE SPACE, AND THE ADAPTIVE POSSIBLE

The potential for variation in outcome in development was first identified by Kacser and Waddington (1957) who introduced the concept of epigenetics and the 'epigenetic landscape'. Kacser and Waddington compared the development and differentiation of a stem cell to the movement of a ball at the top of a hill with different slopes and valleys: as the ball rolls down the hill it will move through different paths until finally reaching a stable situation. They suggested that this concept could be used to consider increasing differentiation of the stem cell on the way to the end state of a fully differentiated cell.

More recently, this concept has become incorporated into discussion about cell differentiation in terms of the concept of the gene regulatory network (Huang 2010). In this approach, rather than linear pathways with gene A resulting in outcome B, the development of a cell is considered to be a result of the combination of the interactions of all the genes within the network. Rather than a linear pathway, a cell is considered to occupy a 'state space' which is a position in a multidimensional space which includes all possible outcomes of the combined interactions of the genes in the network. The interaction of these genes results in changes in the cell and a corresponding change in the cell's state space; this change can be viewed as a trajectory within state space. We discussed this earlier in the context of the output of a system such as an orchestra, namely the music we hear, which we saw can be viewed as a trajectory in a multidimensional space, whose axes or dimensions are defined by all of the variables exerting an influence over the system's current state and on its evolution in time (Schiavio, Maes, and van der Schyff 2021).

When the gene regulatory network is viewed in this way, the dynamics of a system (or interactions) are seen to be more important than the topology of the system (or map of the connections). This may seem confusing until we appreciate that every gene in the network may vary its expression level; at the simplest level, we could imagine each gene as either being 'turned on' or 'turned off'. A network of genes could be imagined as a network of electric bulbs with different patterns seen depending on which bulbs are lighting even though the arrangement of the bulbs does not change. In a biological system, cells will typically move to a space state where they are stable in terms of gene interaction; these positions within the state space are termed 'attractors'. These positions could be considered in terms of Waddington's epigenetic landscape as different valleys into which the ball is likely to roll. The differentiation of a stem cell may thus represent a particular stable state or attractor for the cell (Huang 2010). The state spaces from which a cell is likely to move to a particular attractor are termed the 'basin of attraction' of the attractor. In terms of Waddington's model, these could represent all points from which the ball could roll into a particular valley. Huang suggested that the organisation we find in complex biological systems and the diversity of cell types may not be related to an active process but may instead reflect the response of each cell to gene-expression configurations; in the words of Kauffman, the diversity and organisation of cell types may be 'order for free' (Kauffman 1993).

Although Waddington first used the term 'epigenetic landscape', the concept of development as occurring within a landscape consisting of peaks and valleys (the 'fitness landscape') was first suggested by Wright in 1932 as a way of looking at evolution (Wright 1932). He illustrated the outcome of interaction between genes within a population as resulting in increased fitness (a peak) or decreased fitness (a valley). This concept was extended to the concept of self-organisation and specialisation within complex systems by Kauffman who introduced the concept of the 'adaptive possible' (Kauffman 1993). This reflected the range of possible options available to a system at any point, in the same way that a walker or climber within such a landscape would have particular options to climb further depending on their position. Kauffman discussed the possibility of an organism or species reaching a local peak and being unable to progress further by climbing, in the same way that a climber reaching a smaller peak will not be able to climb any higher to the main peak without first descending the smaller peak. Kauffman and others also discussed the concept of system criticality; this involves the concept of a balance within a complex system between a fixed state and chaos. This position of balance allows a system to be responsive to relatively small stimuli and to adapt optimally to a changing situation or environment.

CONSIDERING MUSCULOSKELETAL GROWTH AS A TRAJECTORY

We have discussed complex systems, organisation of systems, trajectories in state space, system criticality, epigenetic landscapes, the adaptive possible, and entropy. How is all

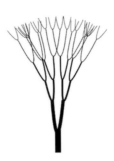

Figure 4.1 Potential trajectories of development of a system.

this relevant to the clinical management of musculoskeletal deformity in children with cerebral palsy? Waddington's epigenetic landscape and the concept of state space and trajectories of growth and development could be used as a metaphor for system development as well as cell development. This concept would apply to the skeleton as well as to skeletal muscle; we could, for example, consider the development of the hip joint in a child with cerebral palsy in this manner. Rather than hip development resulting in either typical development or hip dislocation, there is a range of potential outcomes with a normal hip at one extreme and a dislocated hip at the other. These could be viewed as possible pathways within a branching diagram, analogous to the valleys suggested by Waddington in his epigenetic landscape.

In theory, all outcomes are possible at the outset; as hip development is likely to be a nonlinear process small initial changes are likely to result in different outcomes, represented in Figure 4.1 by a branching diagram. A hip may go on to develop in a typical manner or may go on to become dislocated. As the hip progresses along a particular pathway or trajectory, the range of possible outcomes decrease. It may not be possible in the younger child to predict how a hip will develop, and hips that appear to be showing similar patterns of development may have divergent outcomes. This can be seen clinically in the limited ability of the hip migration index to predict future hip development in children under 8 years with cerebral palsy (Cooke, Cole, and Carey 1989).

We could view a complex system such as a hip joint or skeletal muscle, or indeed a child, as having possible development options within an overall developmental state space; this could be done by extending the earlier diagram as shown in Figure 4.2. The volume within the cone represents potential outcomes at the start of development.

In Chapter 3, we discussed the concept of skeletal muscle not just as a structure but as a process or system resulting from the interaction of complex subsystems including the contractile proteins, sarcoplasmic reticulum, mitochondria, and nucleus. The current state of this system reflects the previous interactions in the system and constrains or influences the subsequent direction of the process. If we wanted to consider the ways in which we can look at or quantify system development and growth we can use the concept of 'thermodynamical depth' which was discussed in Chapter 3 (Lloyd and Pagels 1988). Thermodynamical depth describes the evolution of a state rather than the state itself, and is defined as 'the amount of information required to specify the trajectory that the system

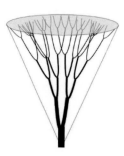

Figure 4.2 Developmental trajectories of a system considered as a cone in state space (see text for discussion).

has followed to its present state'. If we add thermodynamical depth to the axes discussed in the previous chapter, namely algorithmic information content, which reflects the degree of randomness, and 'dynamical depth', which looks at the degree of interactions within a system, we can look at how a system has developed and potentially at what developmental trajectories may be available (Fig. 4.3).

Of note, the discussion of a three-dimensional state space in the context of hip development is for illustration only; a biological state space is likely to have many more dimensions and they are unlikely to be conveniently orthogonal!

If we were to consider hip development in this context we would see a hip joint as occupying a specific state which has been reached through a particular trajectory.

It is possible that hip dislocation and typical hip development may represent relatively stable outcomes or attractor states within the overall context of hip development. In the same way, a skeletal muscle may follow a particular growth trajectory within an available space, and the future trajectory of muscle growth and development will be constrained by the current state of the muscle, which will in turn reflect changes related to earlier development.

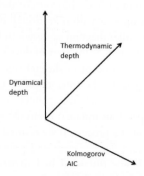

Figure 4.3 Possible axes for a developmental state space (see text for discussion). AIC, algorithmic information content.

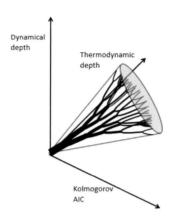

Figure 4.4 Developmental trajectories of the hip joint within a possible developmental state space. AIC, algorithmic information content.

ENTROPY AND DEVELOPMENTAL TRAJECTORIES

The reader may well ask why the developmental outcomes shown above are constrained. The answer to this may lie with the concept of entropy, which we discussed in the previous chapter. As a child develops, the child as an overall complex adaptive system (composed of nested individual complex adaptive systems) becomes more ordered and their overall entropy could be said to decrease. This reduction in entropy, or increase in information, needs an appropriate interaction between the systems involved and enough energy to drive the process and to support the synthesis and organisation of proteins, cell membranes, and other cellular organelles. We will see in the next section how the degree of information (or increase in organisation) in a muscle and in a muscle cell increases with growth. We will consider, for example, the relative immaturity of the contractile proteins, mitochondria, and motor endplates in neonatal muscle as opposed to adult muscle. Skeletal muscle in a neonate can be seen as having higher entropy or less information in comparison to mature skeletal muscle. Neonatal skeletal muscle does have reduced entropy relative to the external environment, but this entropy needs to be lowered further during growth. In a similar manner, the nerves, and bones with which a muscle interacts also need to increase in complexity and organisation with growth, as do the connections and interactions between muscles, bones, and nerves. We can see that growth is thus not simply an increase in size of an organ system but also involves an increase in information and a reduction in entropy together with an increase in system interactions through increased interconnectivity. The capacity for self-organisation may be inherent in complex systems, but the process costs energy, which has to be provided by the cell. A change in trajectory outside of what is possible would not only require energy to reduce the entropy further but would also require energy to reverse the developmental changes that had already occurred to bring the system back to a point in development where an alternative pathway was possible.

An analogy would be an aircraft flight: an aircraft taking off from an airport in London to fly to New York will have a range of possible destinations, constrained by available fuel and by the flight plans. If the flight plans are changed and a new destination such as Rome is announced just after take-off, this will be achievable with mild modifications as it will still be within the list of destinations which could be reached. If a change in the flight plan were to be made when the aircraft is midway across the Atlantic ocean, this would no longer be an achievable destination as it would not only mean flying to Rome from London but also returning to London first. The energy or fuel available to power the aircraft, together with the location of the aircraft, will limit the available destinations.

This concept of constraints on what can be achieved in terms of development is similar to Kauffman's 'adaptive possible', which we discussed above. In the clinical setting, the term 'plasticity' (from the Greek plastikos, able to be moulded) is frequently used in relation to children with cerebral palsy, often in relation to neural tissue where it may involve the perception of a marked capacity for change, including a return to what would be considered as normal. Plasticity, in the sense of the capacity for altered development of any tissue, will be constrained by prior development and by available energy resources. Where we are and where we are going are inevitably influenced by where we have been. The challenge within a complex system is how we predict where we are going. The closer we come to the completion of development, the more accurate we can be in terms of prediction of outcome (although there is still some variability) but the less effective in theory may be any intervention to alter the developmental pathway. In practice, there is no evidence to show that we can positively alter the trajectory of musculoskeletal development and function in a child with cerebral palsy outside of its likely pre-existing range of potential outcomes. This has implications for intervention in terms of treatment aims and goals, which we will discuss in the last chapter.

THIS ALL SOUNDS A BIT COMPLICATED …

This is a different way of looking at the musculoskeletal system and it can initially be a little difficult to see how we could use this approach in a practical way. One way is to construct simple models of the musculoskeletal system which allow us to consider interactions while accepting that these are models or abstractions of reality. When considering biological systems and processes in humans we need to range in size from the proton to the person, which involves 10^{15} orders of magnitude. For illustration, the magnitude of the difference between the dimensions of a proton and the size of our body is similar to the difference between the size of our body and the distance travelled by light in a year (9.5×10^{15} metres). As we move from the person to the proton, we experience further detail and complexity at each level. This means that unlike fractal patterns such as the Mandelbrot set, where we can essentially magnify or zoom in more closely and see the same details repeated endlessly (termed scale-invariance), in a biological system we see instead what is termed a deep 'scale space' with feature richness at multiple levels between systems. As we zoom back out, we can see that each part of the system has properties which would not be obvious from the properties of its component parts and has interactions not present at smaller scales; this feature of complex biological systems, as we have discussed earlier, is termed emergence (Huang and Wikswo 2006). The complexity in biological systems applies to time as well as space: an electron transfer during oxidative phosphorylation takes place in 10^{-15} seconds and contributes to a movement which may be measured in seconds. This range also involves 10^{15} orders of magnitude; to illustrate this we could say that comparing 10^{-15} seconds to 1 second would be similar to comparing 1 second to 10^{15} seconds, which would involve a time interval around 10 million times longer than the time elapsed since the beginning of the universe. This means that the use of a model to explore or even consider such complexity is essential and can be effective as long as we remember the limitations of such a model.

CAUSAL LOOP DIAGRAMS

A frequently used approach in constructing a simplified model of a system to express how the components of a system interact is that of causal loop diagrams. A simple system to consider, for example, would be that of a thermostat controlling room temperature (Fig. 4.5).

In this diagram, each component is shown as having a positive effect on another component (where the component affected increases in quantity or effect) or a negative effect (where the component affected decreases in quantity or effect). We can follow the pathway from any point. The heater in a room will raise the room temperature, this will in turn reduce the effect of the thermostat, which activates the heater. The room heater will stop heating the room so the room temperature will decrease. This will have a less inhibitory effect on the thermostat, which will activate the room heater, so the room temperature will rise again. This is known as a negative feedback cycle and results in stabilisation of the room temperature. There may be delays in the system because the heater or the room may take time to heat up or cool down, and as a result the room temperature may oscillate above and below the desired temperature. Negative feedback loops allow control and stability within a system, and are typical of biological systems. If the room temperature increased the thermostat activity, we would instead have a positive feedback loop where the room temperature would progressively increase. Such a system in isolation would be difficult to sustain but would allow a rapid increase in room temperature over a short period. This would be termed a positive feedback cycle. Some biological processes, such as the generation of an action potential in a nerve as discussed earlier in the chapter, involve such positive feedback. Growth in children also involves an overall positive feedback loop.

A causal loop diagram can allow visualisation of a hypothesis regarding the interactions involved in musculoskeletal growth, and can help us to consider ways in which we can influence this growth. As an example, we can use a causal loop diagram to consider the

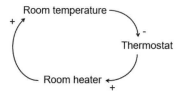

Figure 4.5 A simple causal loop diagram.

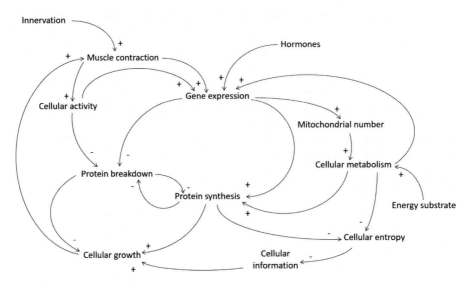

Figure 4.6   A causal loop diagram of myocyte growth.

interactions involved in the growth of a mature muscle cell (discussed in more detail later in the chapter). The factors involved could be visualised as shown in Figure 4.6.

Although this model looks complex at first glance, it considers only a small number of components. It does, however, give an impression of the dynamic nature of the processes involved. The system as modelled has three external inputs, namely innervation, systemic hormones, and an external energy substrate. If we follow the pathway from innervation, we can see that an increase in innervation leads to an increase in muscle contraction, which in turn, through increased gene expression, increases protein synthesis and cellular metabolism resulting in reduced cell entropy and increased muscle cell growth. The concept of entropy was discussed earlier in the chapter; for the purposes of this model it can be considered as a measure of the level of disorganisation within the cell. A reduction in innervation will reduce muscle contraction; this will result in a reduction in protein synthesis and an increase in protein breakdown, which will have a negative effect on muscle cell growth. There are some positive feedback loops in the diagram above; as an example, increased gene expression related to muscle contraction will increase the number of mitochondria present, which will in turn increase the rate of cellular metabolism. This will in turn positively influence gene expression. Ultimately, this is not sustainable but rather than a stable situation which oscillates around a mean, a muscle cell in a child needs to grow and develop so some positive feedback will be necessary. As discussed above, any model by definition will be a simplification of a complex reality so this diagram could be seen as a useful way to consider a system and to consider how inputs to the system affect the output rather than as an exhaustive and detailed description of the system.

Figure 4.6 relates to a single muscle cell; a further causal loop diagram could show how this fits in (or is 'nested') within skeletal muscle as an organ. This model could include contractile tissue such as the muscle cell above, non-contractile tissue such as the connective tissue framework within muscle, and the blood supply and innervation to the muscle. The portion of the model relating to the contractile component of the muscle would need to look at interaction between muscle cells during muscle function and the way in which muscle fibre phenotype (fast or slow muscle) is determined. This model would then need to be nested within a further model which includes the skeletal system and the central nervous system in a way which allows us to consider the interactions involved in musculoskeletal growth and development. The advantage of using a causal loop diagram is that it allows us to look at 'nested' systems, or systems within systems, in a flexible manner which can move to a focus on a specific subsystem or can expand to look at the overall system. We will look at examples of such causal loop diagrams in the next part of the chapter.

ENERGY COSTS OF GROWTH

When considering possible interactions in a developing system, we need also to consider the energy needed for growth. Davies et al. suggested that each gram of body weight gained has an energy density of 5.6kcal (23kJ) (Davies, Ewing, and Lucas 1989). This means that if an infant gained 40g over a 7-day period, this would involve the storage of 224kcal (940kJ). Energy is needed for synthesis of tissues also. Energy costs of protein synthesis have been estimated at 5.5kcal/g, and those of fat synthesis as 1.6kcal/g (Towers et al. 1997). The increased energy costs of protein deposition are likely to include the energy needed to reduce cellular entropy, which for this purpose could be seen as making the cell more organised (this concept is discussed in more detail in Chapter 3).

These energy costs are not uniform within different body organs or tissues. In humans, the main metabolic demand in childhood comes from brain development. Brain development accounts for 52% of resting metabolic requirements (considered to include maintenance functions) at birth in males and 60% in females, decreases during the first 6 months following birth to 37.5% and 41% respectively, and then increases to reach a peak at around the age of 4 years of 66% for males and 65% for females. The increase in glucose use by the brain during the first few years after birth is thought to be related to initial neuronal proliferation and increased connectivity, and subsequent pruning and development with an increased use of anaerobic glycolysis during this time. Following the earlier discussions about interactions within a system, it is perhaps not surprising that brain glucose demand relates inversely to body growth between infancy and puberty suggesting that the high costs of brain development require a compensatory slowing of body growth (Kuzawa et al. 2014). Musculoskeletal growth cannot be considered in isolation but needs to be viewed in the context of energy availability and energy demands throughout the body. Energy availability in neonatal and infant skeletal muscle will also be influenced by the state of development of the mitochondrial network within the muscle cell and the level of development of the enzymes needed for oxidative phosphorylation.

MUSCULOSKELETAL DEVELOPMENT IN THE EMBRYO

We all begin as a fertilised ovum from which the complex tissues and organs that comprise our body, and our musculoskeletal system, develop. Following repeated division of the ovum, the yolk sac and amniotic cavity are formed. Between these two cavities is a thin disc, the epiblast, which will develop into the embryo. For this to happen, the disc has to develop different cell types and to develop a head-tail axis: this process is known as gastrulation.

Most of the information we have about this process comes from the study of mouse and chick embryos (for an excellent discussion see Davies 2014). A structure appears in the tail area of the disc called the primitive streak: this progresses towards the centre as the disc grows in length to become oval. A flat area called the node forms in the centre of the disc: this is followed by proliferation of the cells in the epiblast to form what will become endoderm, the lining of the gut, and to form a structure called the notochord, which will guide the further development of the embryo. The layer of cells which develops between the endoderm and the top layer of the epiblast is called the mesoderm; these cells will give rise to muscles, bones, and tendons. The top layer of the embryo, which was the initial epiblast, becomes ectoderm; this will give rise to skin, hair follicles, pigmented cells, and most of the nervous system.

As the primitive streak forms, part of the ectoderm in what will become the head proliferates and develops to form the neural plate. In what will become the trunk, because of the rate of growth of the embryo and mesoderm, the neural plate forms first a depression and then is enclosed by mesoderm and covered by ectoderm to form the neural tube. Along the side of the neural tube structures called somites form in the mesoderm under the influence of the notochord. These will give rise to the bones and muscles of the trunk and to the muscles of the limbs.

The limbs are formed from small buds, with the upper limb buds forming in humans around 4 weeks after conception and the lower limb buds forming around 2 weeks later. As the limb buds grow, the bones in the limbs form from proximal to distal. Bone can form directly in mesoderm or can form in an existing cartilaginous model. Formation of bone in mesoderm is called intramembranous ossification and is used to form the bones of the skull and the clavicles. Formation of bone in a cartilage model is known as endochondral ossification and forms the pelvis, most of the spine, and the limb bones.

At around 8 postconception weeks (PCW) myoblasts from the somites migrate into the limb buds to form primary myotubes (Ijkema-Paassen and Gramsbergen 2005). The tendons of the developing muscles form in the limb bud as the myotubes form. The migrating myoblasts are accompanied by the growth of αMN axons from the developing spinal cord, which reach and innervate the developing muscles. The primary myoblasts are followed by another wave of myoblasts, which form secondary myotubes. Myoblasts migrating from the somites also give rise to a population of stem cells in muscle, which are termed satellite cells because of their peripheral location on the muscle fibre; these cells will subsequently contribute nuclei to the growing muscle fibres (Schienda et al. 2006). There is limited data available on the types of myosin found in the human fetus. Studies in mice on the expression of MHC suggest that there is a sequential expression of myosin isoforms with a gradual reduction in the amount of developmental (embryonic and perinatal) myosin and an increase in the quantity of adult isoforms, which are mostly expressed post-natally (Agbulut et al. 2003).

MUSCLE CONTRACTION BEGINS EARLY

Muscle contraction is seen in the human between 8PCW and 10PCW (Prechtl 1993) and appears to be caused by intrinsic networks within the developing spinal cord which are capable of ordered discharge without corticospinal or afferent input (Vinay et al. 2002). In the mature musculoskeletal system, as discussed earlier, each muscle fibre is innervated by one αMN; this is termed mononeuronal innervation. In the embryo each muscle fibre may receive input from a number of αMNs; this is termed polyneuronal innervation. In the soleus muscle of the rat, the number of fibres innervating a muscle decreases and mononeuronal innervation occurs just before the rat starts to walk (Ijkema-Paassen and Gramsbergen 2005). We have limited evidence about this process in humans other than a study on the muscle fibres of the psoas muscle, which noted that mononeuronal innervation occurred 12 weeks after birth (Gramsbergen et al. 1997). In humans, sensory fibres from muscles reach the spinal cord by 8PCW and go on to make contact with the αMNs by 9PCW (Clowry 2007). Initially the sensory nerves make abundant connections with neurons across the spinal cord.

THE ROLE OF THE CORTICOSPINAL TRACT

The corticospinal tract appears to have an important role in motor development in the embryo and fetus through trophic effects on the development of intrinsic spinal cord networks (Lemon and Griffiths 2005). Corticospinal tract axons enter the human spinal cord from 17 to 29PCW and innervate the ventral horn from 31 to 35PCW, promoting the development of the intrinsic spinal cord networks, in particular the development of inhibitory interneurons (Clowry 2007). This process is not complete at birth. Martin suggested that refinement of synapses between αMNs, sensory neurons, and interneurons in the spinal cord occur between 1 and 2 years of age in humans and may be related to activity-dependent competition between the neurons involved for synapses within the spinal cord (Martin 2005a). This process results in continued development of the corticospinal tract involving a reduction in the number of neurons in the corticospinal tract, an increase in size of the remaining neurons, and refinement and development of the intrinsic spinal cord networks. This results in an increased duration of innervation of skeletal muscles (Eken, Elder, and Lømo 2008); this is important in terms of function as posture cannot be achieved or maintained unless the muscles involved can maintain a contraction for the necessary duration of the motor activity involved. This process also involves change and development in the neuromuscular junction. In the rat neuromuscular junction, there is a gradual change from low-threshold channels to faster, higher threshold ion channels in mature muscle (Navarrette and Vrbová 1993).

In summary, the interaction of the intrinsic spinal cord networks with the ingrowing corticospinal tract axons appears to facilitate amplification of the corticospinal tract input, development of tonic activation of muscle, maturation of the neuromuscular junction, regression of polyneuronal innervation, and the refinement of afferent input to the spinal cord (Martin 2005b; Clowry 2007; Eken, Elder, and Lømo 2008; Chakrabarty and Martin 2010).

MOVEMENT AND MOTOR CONTROL AFTER BIRTH

The development of movement and motor control continues after birth. Forssberg reviewed human locomotor patterns in infants less than 2 months old, during supported locomotion in older infants 6 to 12 months old, and during early independent walking in infants who were 10 to 18 months old (Forssberg 1985). He suggested that innate pattern generators in the spinal cord produce infant stepping, and generate the basic locomotor rhythm in adults, but that neural circuits specific for humans transform the original, non-plantigrade motor activity to a plantigrade motor pattern. Sutherland et al. noted differences in the activation patterns of muscles in children between the age of 1 and 2 years and reported alteration in the tibialis anterior (prolonged activity in stance), vastus medialis (prolonged activity in swing), and in the gastrocnemius and soleus muscles (prolonged activity beginning near the middle of swing) (Sutherland, Olshen, and Biden 1988). In children aged 4 years a more mature pattern was seen in the majority of the muscles assessed. These changes are likely to be associated with an improvement in the ability of the spinal cord to filter afferent input and to develop reciprocal inhibition. O'Sullivan et al. (1991) noted a gradual increase in the stimulus needed to invoke a monosynaptic reflex in typically developing children, increasing from a low level at birth to an adult level by the age of 6 years.

There appears to be close interaction in the child between the development of motor output and the subsequent development of sensory feedback and integration, with skeletal muscle acting as an essential part of a feedback loop. The development of a cortical motor map in the cat appears to depend on activity and motor experience (Martin 2005a). The refinement of the corticospinal tract of the cat in terms of its connections in the spinal cord, and the integration of afferent fibres from muscle, appear to be driven by movement. Blocking limb use in the cat between 3 and 7 weeks postnatally with the use of botulinum toxin resulted in a persistent abnormal morphology of corticospinal tract axon terminals in the spinal cord and a persistent prehension deficit (Martin 2005b). Clowry et al. noted similar findings in rats following the use of botulinum toxin in the second postnatal week to cause temporary limb paresis and suggested that this may be related to competition between the corticospinal tract axons, muscle afferent fibres, and other inputs for cord synapses (Clowry, Walker, and Davies 2006). Reduced refinement of afferent input terminations in the spinal cord and impaired inhibition because of reduced corticospinal tract input may lead to a continued heightened motor response to afferent input such as a muscle stretch.

If we were to consider these interactions in a causal loop diagram, it could look something like Figure 4.7. The causal loop diagram in Figure 4.6, for skeletal muscle growth could be seen as nested in the lower left-hand corner of this diagram. The input shown as 'innervation' in the earlier diagram has here been expanded to look at development of muscle innervation, and some links have been included to show the interactions with the sensory system.

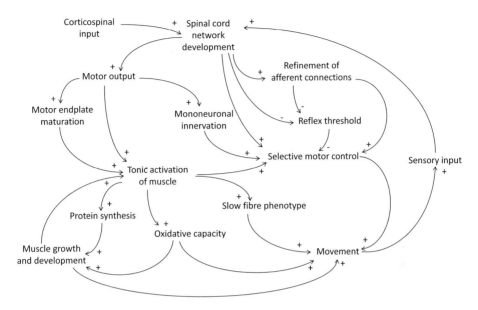

Figure 4.7 Interactive pathways in the development of movement.

As with the earlier diagrams, the interactions shown should not be seen as representing all interactions within a system but instead are selected both to allow clarity and to allow a focus on a particular aspect of a system.

SKELETAL MUSCLE FIBRE GROWTH AND DEVELOPMENT

There is limited information on antenatal human muscle fibre growth and development. Moore et al. reported that the muscle fibres in the sartorius muscle in humans appear to double in diameter between midgestation and term, and Schloon et al. noted an increased growth in overall muscle fibre diameter between 35 weeks gestation and term (Moore et al. 1971; Schloon et al. 1979).

As noted earlier, most muscles have their fibres arranged not in the long axis of the muscle but instead attached to the tendon at an angle called the pennation angle. Because of this, muscle fibres can contribute to growth of the muscle belly through an increase in muscle fibre length and through an increase in muscle fibre diameter. Oertel studied postmortem sections of the human vastus lateralis and deltoid and noted an increase in mean fibre diameter from 10 to 12 microns shortly after birth to 40 to 60 microns between the ages of 15 and 20 years (Oertel 1988). Lexell et al. (1992) noted that the mean fibre diameter of the human vastus lateralis in postmortem specimens doubles between the ages of 5 and 20 years.

Bénard et al. (2011) used ultrasound to study the growth of the medial gastrocnemius in children aged between 5 and 12 years; they were not able to visualise individual muscle fibres and instead assessed muscle fascicle (or fibre bundle) changes with growth.

They found that muscle fascicle length and diameter increase with growth, but because of the pennate nature of the gastrocnemius, longitudinal muscle fascicle growth accounts for only 20% of the longitudinal growth of the medial gastrocnemius muscle belly: the remaining 80% was related to the increase in diameter of the muscle fascicles.

The contribution of muscle fibre growth in length and muscle fibre growth in diameter to longitudinal growth and increased volume of the muscle belly is likely to vary depending on the morphology of individual muscles, but it would seem reasonable to say that muscle belly growth depends as much on muscle fibre growth in diameter as it does in length.

FACTORS INFLUENCING MUSCLE FIBRE GROWTH

Growth and development of muscle fibres is accompanied by growth and organisation of the connective tissue framework within the muscle. Myostatin, which appears to have a role in the maintenance of muscle connective tissue, appears to be suppressed during perinatal and early postnatal muscle growth in rats, possibly to enhance development of the contractile component of muscle (Nishimura et al. 2007).

In the pig, the growth of muscle fibres in late gestation and in the perinatal period appears to be dependent on an adequate supply of amino acids (Brameld et al. 1998). Muscle protein synthesis in neonatal pigs is associated with an increased sensitivity to growth hormones, insulin, and amino acids, and with a marked increase in mitochondrial activity due to an increase in mitochondrial number (Schmidt and Herpin 1997). The increased sensitivity of neonatal muscle to growth hormone, insulin, and amino acids appears to decrease with age (Suryawan et al. 2007). The importance of early nutrition in muscle growth, and the presence of an optimal growth period during which the muscle may show increased responsiveness to endocrine factors and nutrition, is supported by studies on the effect of the timing of nutritional restriction in animal studies. In rats, undernutrition prior to weaning can cause permanent stunting of muscle growth but the effect of undernutrition subsequent to weaning can generally be reversed (Bedi et al. 1982). Muscle growth may be selectively limited in the antenatal or perinatal period if nutrition is impaired. A relative inhibition of fetal skeletal muscle growth has been noted in a sheep model of late placental insufficiency/intrauterine growth restriction (Thorn et al. 2009), suggesting that skeletal muscle growth may be preferentially downregulated if nutrition is compromised at this time.

Muscle fibre development, the metabolic capacity of the muscle fibre, and the development of the connective tissue network of muscle thus appear to reflect the interplay of a number of factors including neuronal, nutritional, and hormonal factors and the initial and subsequent pattern of muscle use. Mouse models of neonatal brachial plexus palsy described above, which involve experimental denervation of a single muscle group in otherwise healthy mice (Kim et al. 2009; Nikolaou et al. 2011) suggest that the pattern of neuronal activation of muscle may be particularly important in postnatal muscle fibre growth and in the development of slow or fast muscle types. The most important factors influencing perinatal and early postnatal muscle growth would thus appear to be the appropriate development of muscle innervation and the energy available for muscle growth.

EFFECT OF SKELETAL MUSCLE ON SKELETAL DEVELOPMENT

Muscles act on the growing skeleton and influence skeletal development in a number of ways. As a bone grows in length, it needs to grow also in diameter if bone strength is to be maintained (Rauch 2005). The factors influencing bone growth are complex but lean body mass appears to be the strongest predictor of total body mineral content (Crabtree et al. 2004). Heinonen et al. showed a significant correlation on magnetic resonance imaging (MRI) between tibial cortical area and muscle cross-sectional area (MCSA) in prepubertal females (Heinonen et al. 2001). MacDonald et al. (2006) found that MCSA was the primary explanatory variable for tibial bone strength and geometry after allowing for tibial length; from their model, an increase in MCSA would lead to an increase in bone strength.

Skeletal muscles also act on a growing bone to influence its shape: the proximal femur is a good example. In the fetal and neonatal femur, the angle between the femoral neck and shaft is much greater than in the adult, so that in the coronal plane the femur is relatively straighter, and anteversion, the degree to which the proximal femur is rotated in the transverse plane, is much greater. Between birth and the age of 7 years, the angle between the femoral neck and femoral shaft gradually reduces to an adult level (Osborne et al. 1980). The angle between the femoral neck and shaft appears to increase, making the proximal femur straighter, in the first year after birth and then begins to gradually decrease at around the time that the child begins to stand and take steps (Morgan and Somerville 1960). This has been attributed to the effect of body weight but modelling of the proximal femur would suggest instead that the alteration in shape is related primarily to the loading imposed on the proximal femur through the greater trochanter by the abductor muscles (Shefelbine and Carter 2004). Using a causal loop diagram, this process can be shown in Figure 4.8 (the developing muscle cell previously discussed would be nested within the input labelled as 'hip abductor muscle growth').

Figure 4.8 has two inputs and has a positive feedback loop (despite the negative signs) leading to an alteration in femoral shape. The development of hip abductor muscle force, which contributes to the ability of the child to stand, is associated with increased growth of the lateral aspect of the proximal femur. An increase in lateral femoral growth relative to medial growth in this model will result in a reduction of the neck shaft angle, which would in turn increase the moment arm (perpendicular distance between the centre of rotation of the joint and the line of action of the abductor muscles) of the hip abductor muscles; this would in turn further reduce the neck shaft angle. Reduced hip abductor muscle growth, from Figure 4.8, would result in persistence of a valgus femoral neck-shaft angle, with altered orientation of the proximal femoral physis and impaired development of both acetabular shape and femoral had position. This causal loop diagram, as in all such diagrams, is a simplified and somewhat selective model of a complex system but does allow a conjectured explanation of why interventions such as bracing, supported standing, or the use of botulinum toxin have not been shown to positively influence hip development in children with cerebral palsy.

In Figure 4.8, 'Standing' appears to have only one input. For the development of a more specific functional movement, such as standing or walking, we need to consider wider aspects of the system. We would need to look at the musculoskeletal system and also

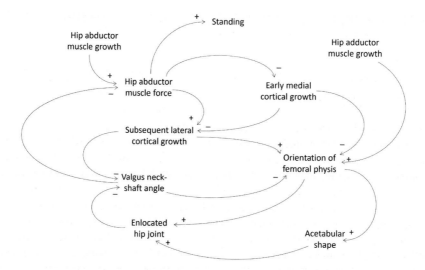

Figure 4.8 Possible interactive pathways in hip joint development.

consider vision, cognition, and balance. We would also need to look at the environment in which the child was developing. Such a diagram may look like Figure 4.9.

The previous figures can be seen within Figure 4.9, but we can also see that what has been termed 'functional walking capacity' is the result of an interaction between the

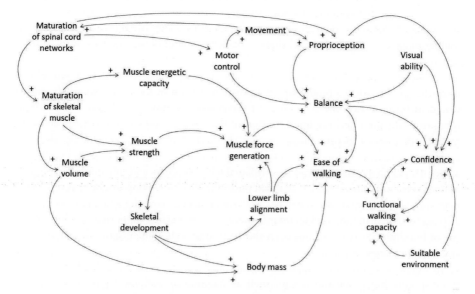

Figure 4.9 Interactive pathways leading to musculoskeletal function.

musculoskeletal system, the central nervous system, cognitive factors such as the level of confidence of the child, and the environment in which they are walking.

MUSCULOSKELETAL DEVELOPMENT IN CHILDREN WITH CEREBRAL PALSY

The interaction between the components of the developing musculoskeletal system, the nonlinearity of the system, and the capacity of the system to adapt and self-organise mean that the effect of an alteration in one aspect of the system on the overall function and development of the system can be difficult to predict. Development of the musculoskeletal system involves interaction and integration between the components or subsystems of the overall system. This means that the musculoskeletal system can be viewed at any time point in development as a process which has developed through previous interactions, and which will continue to develop as the child grows. The musculoskeletal system of a 2-year-old child will be significantly advanced in comparison to how it was when the child was born, but as we have discussed the subsequent development of the system will be influenced by the initial state of the system, by the pattern of interaction of the system elements, by the resulting sensory and motor experience of the child, and by the available energy resources. An alteration in one or more elements of a developing system, or a limitation in available energy, may alter the trajectory of development of the system.

Could the musculoskeletal changes seen in children with cerebral palsy be explained as an altered trajectory of a complex adaptive system? The findings of an early reduction in skeletal muscle volume associated with increased passive muscle stiffness and altered gene expression within the muscle (Barber et al. 2011; Smith et al. 2011; Willerslev-Olsen et al. 2013, 2018) could be viewed in the context of altered interaction of the neuronal, nutritional, and endocrine factors noted above. A reduced input of the corticospinal tract to the developing spinal cord networks, and the resulting impaired development of these networks, would lead to persistence of polyneuronal innervation of muscle fibres, reduced ability to maximally activate muscle fibres, impaired development of motor endplates, impaired development of the tonic activation of muscle needed for development and growth of slow muscle fibres, and impaired development of posture and ambulation. A reduction in muscle fibre diameter will affect muscle belly length because of the pennate nature of skeletal muscle; a reduced rate of muscle fibre hypertrophy with growth may thus present clinically as progressive shortness of the muscle belly. The metabolic capacity of skeletal muscle will also be influenced by impairment of muscle innervation resulting in reduced muscle oxidative capacity and mitochondrial biogenesis (Schiaffino, Sandri, and Murgia 2007; Westerblad, Bruton, and Katz 2010). This may in part explain the impaired mitochondrial function reported in the muscles of children with cerebral palsy (Dayanidhi et al. 2021). Some studies on gene expression in the muscles of children with cerebral palsy (Smith et al. 2009, 2012) show upregulation of some cellular processes and downregulation of other processes, but these do not appear to be consistent between muscles. Smith et al. (2012), looking at hamstring muscles in children with cerebral palsy and in typically developing children, reported a downregulation of genes related to muscle metabolism, and noted a significant negative correlation between muscle stiffness and expression of a gene related to mitochondrial structure. These muscle samples were taken from children undergoing surgery, and may reflect a combination of an endpoint of a particular developmental trajectory and the effect of previous interventions.

If we consider cerebral palsy as an emergent property of altered interactions within a complex adaptive system, this allows us to include factors other than altered innervation which may also influence early musculoskeletal growth and development. The energy needed for cell growth and development in the fetus and infant, as discussed above, needs to be met from the energy sources available; this essentially depends on a combination of energy substrate availability and on mitochondrial number and function. We saw earlier that cells allow growth and development when energy is freely available, and limit growth if there is limited available energy. We generally consider the neurological deficit as being the primary cause of cerebral palsy, with alteration in muscle growth and skeletal growth seen as secondary changes resulting from the neurological deficit. It is possible that in some cases the neurological insult leading to the clinical picture of cerebral palsy may result from a significant impairment in energy availability to the developing body as a whole. This may be seen most in the central nervous system because of the significant metabolic demands involved, but the global lack of available energy may also adversely affect muscle development in a way which is subsequently exacerbated by the altered neurological development.

Children born preterm may have impaired muscle growth because of nutritional causes (Hay and Thureen 2010), and impaired or limited early nutrition may result in a preferential downregulation of skeletal muscle growth (Thorn et al. 2009). The effects of energy substrate availability on gene expression and cell growth may be mediated through histone acetylation and DNA methylation as discussed earlier. Skeletal myoblast differentiation in mice, for example, is inhibited by glucose restriction through activation of sirtuins through the AMPK pathway (Fulco et al. 2008). The combination of impaired muscle activation due to altered development of muscle innervation, and impaired muscle cell growth and differentiation related to impaired nutrition during this time, may result in reduced sensitivity to, or failure of, the accelerated muscle development which typically occurs in the last trimester and in infancy. This in turn may be exacerbated by the presence of sepsis or inflammation in the perinatal period, which may alter the balance between growth of contractile and non-contractile material within the muscle through enhancement of the action of myostatin (Nishimura et al. 2007; Zhu et al. 2007; Kollias and McDermott 2008; Menconi et al. 2010); the use of steroids during this period may further impair early muscle growth (Menconi et al. 2010). These mechanisms could explain the reduced size of skeletal muscle in children with cerebral palsy from an early age (Willerslev-Olsen et al. 2018).

EFFECT OF EARLY DEVELOPMENTAL CHANGES ON SUBSEQUENT MUSCULOSKELETAL GROWTH AND DEVELOPMENT

The alteration in early muscle development in children with cerebral palsy has consequences for subsequent skeletal muscle growth and development. Children with cerebral palsy have been shown to have reduced numbers of satellite cells, with reduced myogenic potential, which is related to methylation of DNA (Domenighetti et al. 2018). Impaired development of the innervation of skeletal muscle, a reduction in satellite cell number, and a persistent alteration in muscle gene expression due to the epigenetic factors discussed would result in a continued impairment of muscle growth, development, and function in children with cerebral palsy. Von Walden et al. noted reduced numbers of satellite cells in skeletal muscle of children with cerebral palsy together with increased inflammatory markers associated with increased collagen synthesis and increased myostatin expression (Von Walden et al. 2018). They also noted suppression of muscle ribosome biogenesis, which would further reduce the ability of the muscle to synthesis the proteins needed for cell growth. An imbalance between the growth of contractile and noncontractile tissue in the skeletal muscle of children with cerebral palsy may explain the increased resting sarcomere lengths in the semitendinosus in children with cerebral palsy in the presence of increased connective tissue (Smith et al. 2011). Increased resting sarcomere lengths in the gastrocnemius and soleus muscles may contribute (along with other factors discussed below) to an equinus gait pattern, as the active length of a muscle will need to be shorter than the passive length if sufficient force is to be generated to allow walking.

Muscle injury due to altered loading in the presence of reduced numbers of satellite cells and reduced ribosome capacity may lead to fibrosis and replacement of muscle fibres by fat, which is seen in older children and adults with cerebral palsy (Serrano and Muñoz-Cánoves 2010; Noble et al. 2014). To understand how injury may lead to fibrosis and fat infiltration, it may be helpful to consider the processes involved in the repair of an injured muscle fibre (Dort et al. 2019). Injury to a muscle fibre results in macrophage activation, with monocytes from the circulation promoting an initial inflammatory response which acts to clear cellular debris. The monocytes then seem to promote an anti-inflammatory response; this leads to activation of stem cells called fibroadipogenic progenitors (FAPs), which can develop into fibroblasts or adipose cells. The FAPs in turn activate muscle stem cells, which respond by suppressing the FAPs and forming myotubes which develop into regenerated skeletal muscle. Persisting inflammation will prevent the monocyte-orchestrated shift from a pro-inflammatory response to an anti-inflammatory response, and in this way will impair healing; a reduction in muscle stem cells will prevent regeneration of muscle and FAP inhibition resulting in fibrofatty repair instead of myocyte regeneration.

Rather than a single mechanism or pathway leading to altered muscle development in all children with cerebral palsy, there may be different pathways depending on the interaction between the severity of the initial insult, the extent of neurological injury, perinatal sepsis and inflammation, subsequent muscle use, and clinical intervention. Fibrosis and fatty change in the muscles of ambulant children, for example, may be related to overuse and chronic injury, while fatty changes and fibrosis in non-ambulant children may be related more to impaired early muscle development because of reduced innervation. Altered innervation postnatally may result in reduced mitochondrial biogenesis and in suppression of muscle growth through the AMPK pathway and through impaired ribosome synthesis as discussed earlier. In the presence of an adequate nutritional intake, impaired muscle protein synthesis may result in the energy being stored instead as fat. An imbalance between the amount of adipose tissue and skeletal muscle tissue in the body could further alter the interaction between these tissues as noted earlier and in this way inhibit muscle growth.

A reduction in skeletal muscle mitochondrial function and in energy availability could also in theory impair muscle function in a manner which could explain the clinical features ascribed to 'spasticity'. We generally consider skeletal muscles as 'relaxed' or 'active' but the entropy, or disorder, in a skeletal muscle will be highest during contraction and will be lowest when the muscle is ready for contraction when the myocyte and its components are in their most ordered and predictable state (Christlieb and Cesarman 1996). Restoring this order after muscle contraction will require an input of energy as the tendency of the muscle will be to move to a state of higher entropy. It may be more economical in terms of energy balance for a muscle to maintain a continuous low-grade contraction than it is to 'reset' all of the cellular mechanisms following contraction. This is not to suggest that neural mechanisms are not involved but instead to suggest that other mechanisms may also be involved.

Altered muscle development in children with cerebral palsy could in turn explain the development of skeletal deformities in these children. Hip dysplasia occurs in children with cerebral palsy, with an increased incidence of hip dysplasia with increased functional impairment of the child (Soo et al. 2006). This is often attributed to spasticity but may instead be related to altered early development of the proximal femur due to an altered pattern of muscle loading, particularly from the hip abductor muscles. Consideration of the hip joint as a complex system in itself would explain the difficulty in predicting the natural history of hip dysplasia and the likely outcome of intervention in an individual (Cooke, Cole, and Carey 1989); if typical hip development and a dislocated hip are seen as suggested earlier as attractors within a system this could explain the trajectory of a hip towards typical development or dysplasia. Children with cerebral palsy have an increased risk of fracture of the long bones of the lower limb; although this has been attributed to osteoporosis, this diagnosis has often been based on dual energy X-ray absorptiometry, which gives an estimate of bone volume based on a measure of bone area, and which as a result may significantly underestimate bone density in smaller bones (Specker and Schoenau 2005). More accurate assessment of bone density in children with cerebral palsy using peripheral quantitative computed tomography (Binkley et al. 2005) or MRI (Modlesky et al. 2009; Noble et al. 2014) showed that bone density in children with cerebral palsy is similar to that of typically developing children, but bone cross-sectional area and hence bone strength is reduced. The reduction in cross-sectional muscle area and muscle volume in the thigh may explain the reduction in femoral cross-sectional area in ambulant children and young people with cerebral palsy (Noble et al. 2014).

Consideration of the musculoskeletal system as part of a feedback loop involving the integration of motor output, limb movement, and sensory feedback may also help us to consider the importance of sensory development. Movement-associated refinement of the afferent connections may contribute to the reduction in the threshold for stretch reflex seen with typical motor development (Gibson and Clowry 1999). The sensory feedback from movement also appears to contribute to development of sensory and motor representation in the cerebral cortex (Chakrabarty and Martin 2000; Martin, Engber, and Meng 2005). In the adult animal, a reduction of limb use through immobilisation may adversely affect both the cortical sensory map (Coq and Xerri 1999) and the cortical motor map (Liepert, Tegenthoff, and Malin 1995). There is limited information as yet about sensory development in children with cerebral palsy. Wingert et al. (2010) found reduced but much more diffuse cortical activation in response to sensory input to the finger of children with cerebral palsy in comparison to typically developing children. Hoon et al. (2009) used diffusion tensor imaging to assess the corticospinal tract and posterior thalamocortical radiation of children with cerebral palsy born preterm. They described abnormalities of both pathways but noted that posterior thalamic radiation injury correlated with sensory and motor involvement, whereas corticospinal tract injury did not correlate with motor or sensory outcome measures.

Altered sensory development in children with cerebral palsy is often not considered, possibly because quantitative measurement is not straightforward, but may contribute to phenomena we see in children with cerebral palsy such as toe-walking which may provide increased stability in the presence of reduced proprioceptive input from the limbs. Lorentzen at al. suggested that an equinus gait in children with cerebral palsy may be related to the interaction of a number of factors including altered muscle morphology as noted earlier and persistence of agonist/antagonist cocontraction (Lorentzen et al. 2019). They suggested that the resulting increased stiffness of the limb may compensate for the lack of feed-forward motor control discussed earlier, for reduced sensory and motor signal-to-noise rations, and for reduced muscle strength by reducing the degree of control needed in terms of joint motion during gait.

PUTTING IT ALL TOGETHER: UNDERSTANDING AND EXPLORING THE MUSCULOSKELETAL SYSTEM

The musculoskeletal system has been presented as a complex adaptive system and the integration and interdependence of the different parts of the system have been discussed. The altered musculoskeletal development seen in children with cerebral palsy can be considered as an emergent property of a complex adaptive system due to an altered trajectory of development. The interaction between the components of the system, the nonlinearity of the system as a whole, and the capacity of the system to adapt and self-organise mean that the effect of an alteration in one aspect of the system on overall system development and function can be difficult to predict. As an example, if we look at the causal loop diagram shown earlier (Figure 4.6) for skeletal muscle cell growth, we can see by following the pathways of interactions from the innervation input in the top left of Figure 4.6 that a reduction in innervation (shown by a dashed line rather than a solid line) will affect all of the pathways (Fig. 4.10).

In a similar manner, however, if the energy substrate input or the hormonal input is reduced in Figure 4.10, we would also see widespread effects through the system. Which of these external factors have priority? We could hypothesise from the evidence available from the outcome of botulinum toxin injections in healthy and well-nourished animals noted earlier (Kim et al. 2009; Nikolaou et al. 2011) that innervation of muscle has priority. If we wanted to investigate this experimentally, a causal loop diagram can act as the visualisation of a hypothesis which can inform investigation. The interactions and interrelationship of the elements of the causal loop diagram can also make us cautious about inferring or assuming causality. As is often discussed in statistics courses, the close correlation between ice cream sales and number of drownings does not, unfortunately, mean that banning ice cream sales would result in a reduction in the number of people who drown; there is an underlying confounding variable, namely temperature, which influences both ice cream

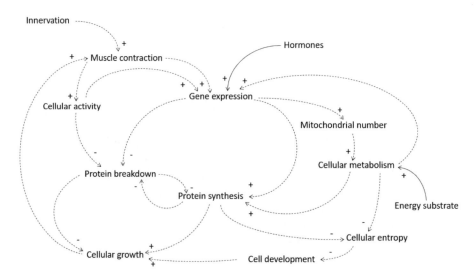

Figure 4.10   Muscle developmental pathways which may be altered or impaired in children with cerebral palsy.

sales and the number of people who go swimming. Awareness of interactions within a system can help us to identify such confounding variables.

The use of causal loop diagrams allows us to understand how intervention in a child with cerebral palsy to alter a specific component of the system, particularly a structural component, may have a limited impact on the overall function of the system. If we take, for example, the effect of surgery to improve lower limb alignment on the capacity of a child with cerebral palsy to walk, we could look at the system node entitled 'lower limb alignment' and its connections as shown in the diagram below on walking (Fig. 4.11). We can see that alteration of lower limb alignment in isolation may have a limited impact on function (shown by the dashed lines) and that for an optimal effect we would also need to consider whether intervention to improve muscle force generation, balance, and confidence is possible, and also consider the environment in which the child is walking. In a similar manner, if we look at Figure 4.8 on proximal femoral development we can see that surgery to alter the valgus neck shaft angle of the proximal femur may be associated with a subsequent recurrence of a valgus neck shaft angle if there is persistently impaired hip abductor muscle growth.

WHERE DO WE GO FROM HERE?

Causal loop diagrams are useful tools which can help the development and visualisation of hypotheses regarding interactions within a system, and in this way help suggest portals through which the development of the system can be influenced. Use of these models to inform clinical practice offers both challenges and opportunities and will involve quantification of the strength of the interactions involved and an understanding of how these

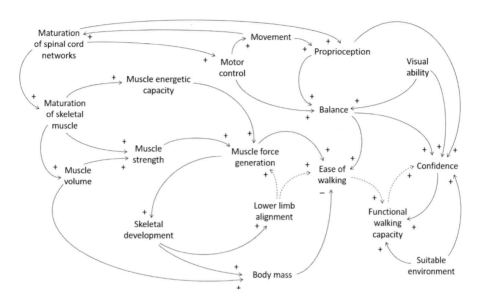

Figure 4.11   Impact of surgery to improve limb alignment in the context of other pathways influencing function in the child with cerebral palsy.

interactions may vary between individuals. As an example, we could consider an equinus gait in a child with cerebral palsy. This may be (and often is) viewed as a pathological entity related to spasticity but this does not advance clinical management. If we see an equinus gait instead as the output of a system we can begin to look at the underlying processes. From the discussions above, an equinus gait could be related to a need to avoid stretch on overlong sarcomeres and in this way maintain sarcomere length at an optimal level for force production, it could be related to reduced capacity to develop a low-entropy state in muscle because of impaired energy availability, and it could be related to a need to provide increased stability in the presence of reduced proprioception. It is thus likely that an equinus gait may have different underlying processes and different interactions of these processes in different children meaning that the same clinical approach for all children with an equinus gait will not be effective. This will be discussed in the next chapter where we will consider the limited degree to which we can apply data from population studies to the clinical management of an individual child, and where we will discuss how we view and define 'causation'.

The concept of the musculoskeletal system of a child with cerebral palsy as a complex adaptive system with an altered trajectory of development offers both challenges and opportunities. It allows us to focus on molecular interactions within the cell and on the interaction of the child and their environment, while seeing both of these as parts of the same overall process. It does however move away from the apparent simplicity and attractiveness of the present model and would seem to replace certainty with uncertainty. How we deal with this, and how we can consider this approach in the context of the lived experience of the child with cerebral palsy will be discussed in the last chapter.

Evidence-Based Medicine and Cerebral Palsy

José is a football-mad 10-year-old boy with cerebral palsy. He goes to the same school as his identical twin, Brendan, but he struggles to be included in the activities that his brother does. He is aware of the stark differences between his brother's experiences of school and his own, struggling to be included in the same playground activities, having a smaller social grouping, and not participating in the after-school football club. He thinks that it is unfair that his body has grown differently to Brendan's and wonders why that is. He has started to read about cerebral palsy on the Internet, and is drawn to the claims of certain doctors and therapists who propose curative treatments. These are in contrast to the opinions of his own doctors, who advise managing the decline of his condition, and are enthusiastic about providing assistive technology. He is confused by the mixed messages, and angry that there appear to be options out there for him that he is denied.

At some point in their childhood, children may gain a greater awareness of their disability, making comparisons between their lives and those of their peers. In a world where science and technology has made such great advances, and modern medicine has kept people living for longer, defied mortal diseases, and transformed the quality of many lives. It may appear to these children that they have been left behind; that in some way they matter less than others.

Dr Maria Saint-Vincent is a molecular biologist working in cancer research. Recently, she has been part of a large well-funded team engaged in understanding and developing new therapies for the treatment of pancreatic cancer. The team are well thought of, and many of their peers believe that Maria and her colleagues are on the verge of a significant breakthrough in this area.

Great advances in the treatment of childhood cancer and asthma have been made in recent decades, and new and promising therapies are being developed all the time.

Maria has a nephew, José, with cerebral palsy. She has watched closely over the years how José has developed. She has seen how his muscles have become tighter and how his limbs appear twisted. She has often pondered on the origins of his musculoskeletal problems and on the therapies that might be available to treat them. Her brother, Manuel, has told Maria that the family are discussing management options for José with their orthopaedic specialist. On exploring the literature, Maria finds that the interventions available for José are crude, even primitive. She wonders why there is so little biological explanation of the development of neurological problems and of musculoskeletal deformity. She is not surprised though that, with so little understanding of deformity, the treatments on offer have only moderate effect sizes.

> **Current interventions in cerebral palsy are blunt instruments. They treat the results of complex biological processes at the level of the limb rather than probing and addressing the mechanisms themselves.**
>
> Jen is a young academic physiotherapist who used to review José, but has moved on to take a part-time role at a local university. She has just completed a Cochrane review in stretch casting in young children with mild to moderate plantarflexion. She was surprised at the paucity of high-level evidence to support the practice. Surprised because her clinical peers have always claimed that for the right child stretch casting can alleviate muscle shortness, maintain muscle length in the long term, and delay orthopaedic surgery.
>
> **The experience of the practitioner does not always match the results of the research trial. Why do disparities between the evidence and the clinical experience exist? How in the future might these disparities be resolved?**
>
> Manuel Fields is the father of twins, aged 10 years, José and Brendan. He has closely watched how the twins have developed. José and Brendan were born preterm, and while Brendan has developed typically, José's development has taken a different path with the development of muscular and bony problems. He wonders how two children, raised so similarly, can grow to be so different, and which factors have influenced these diverse trajectories. Manuel reflects on the boys' futures and wonders if José's trajectory might be improved, so that he might have an adult life comparable to his brother's.
>
> **The person with cerebral palsy may have problems dealing with adult life. They may live in pain. They may develop cardiometabolic conditions that are life-shortening and difficult to manage. Employment rates are low among individuals with cerebral palsy and participation in marriage and parenting very limited. Some of these issues are associated with level of ambulatory mobility. Presently, we know little of the effect of our interventions on the long-term outcomes, and it is possible that treatments proposed to improve mobility in childhood do not positively affect long-term development and maintenance of physical function, and the quality of life of the adult.**

In this chapter, we will contrast the spectacular advances made in several areas of paediatric medicine in the last three decades with the slower progress made in cerebral palsy. We will discuss alternative ways of creating knowledge to inform our clinical practices. We will construct a model of functional ability across the lifespan to help us understand the effect of interventions made in children, on mobility in adulthood. We will discuss methods that improve the strength of our scientific claims.

CLINICAL EXPERIENCE AND EVIDENCE-BASED MEDICINE

In each episode of the long-running television series *House*, Dr House (played by the British actor Hugh Laurie) would encounter an extraordinary clinical case. This grumpy doctor would snarl at the fruitless efforts of his colleagues to diagnose and treat the patient. Eventually, after a number of clinical investigations, some failed treatments, a lot of coffee and illicit prescription drugs, and the exercising of an incredible mind, Dr House would save the day (and the patient). Every one of the 790 episodes had a similar narrative but were, nonetheless, enjoyable.

We have all come across instances when an experienced clinician who makes a diagnosis, and gives an intuitive and correct decision after limited contact with the patient. What they are doing is relying on a wealth of experience and an ability to make associations between the symptoms displayed, the patient's underlying condition, and their knowledge of the available treatments. Often this works very well, but there will be times when an individual clinician has a problem which is beyond their associative abilities and their experience. There will be challenges to their associative power when previous decisions that they have made were *potentially* incorrect, *potentially* resulting in some bad outcome for a patient. It is the human condition to invent worlds which never existed. These alternative universes are created by the 'What if?' proposition. For example, what if I had not intervened? Would the patient's trajectory have been better? These counterfactuals invoke emotions in the clinician including doubt and regret. In fact, we understand that recent experiences, particularly bad ones, have a disproportionate impact on our powers of association. Experience is useful but bad experiences can lead us to doubt our decision-making abilities, drive us to become risk adverse, and to make wrong decisions in the future. A clinician with doubts may consult with their colleagues but their advice may be tainted with their own regrets, biases, and misunderstandings.

Evidence-based medicine (EBM) (Sackett et al. 1996) has emerged as an alternative paradigm in which high-quality evidence, clinical experience, and patient preferences combine to deliver better decision-making. Evidence is obtained principally through clinical trials and meta-analyses of trial data and findings. Clinicians are encouraged to place the available evidence in the context of their experience and their patients' preferences. However, how this works in practice is unclear. There are a few instances in medicine where a new treatment is so overwhelmingly superior to the standard treatment that the strict adherence to guidelines based on the evidence from trials should be mandatory. Most trials do not suggest 100% efficacy for a new treatment. Usually, there is some room for doubt with certain individuals from the group receiving the standard treatment seeming to have better outcomes than in the novel treatment group. How does the physician, surgeon, or physiotherapist decide to treat the *individual* patient when the intervention recommended by a guideline has only been shown to work on *average*? It is true that often subgroup analyses are conducted in which the response to a group of patients with particular characteristics are evaluated, but many trials do not have the necessary statistical power to do so. Do clinicians in general feel able to contradict the guideline and use their understanding of the patient to propose an alternative treatment? Do they have the confidence to defend their position if the treatment does not work out for the patient? Even if they felt confident, they might find it difficult to articulate their defence if their understanding was tacit or based on previous experience.

There is no doubt that EBM had been a positive influence on outcomes for patients with many conditions, but where heterogeneity exists in the characteristics of a population and in their responses to treatment, and when the treatments themselves only produce moderate average improvements, we should be more circumspect about applying trial results and recommendations from guidelines.

THE PROBLEM WITH RANDOMISED CONTROLLED TRIALS IN CEREBRAL PALSY

In 2013, Novak et al. (2013) published an analysis of systematic reviews, and other sources of evidence, in the area of treatment in cerebral palsy. Each systematic review was an analysis of the controlled trials and other studies in a particular area. Novak et al.'s article is both comprehensive in its coverage of the evidence at the time, and highly influential, being the most downloaded article in the history of the journal where it was published. The authors used the Grading of Recommendations, Assessment, Development, and Evaluations (GRADE) system of judging research quality and potential impact (Irvine et al. 2002). GRADE assesses the research in two ways.

1. The quality of the evidence presented in the research, in other words the level of certainty that one can attribute to the findings. This may depend on the risk of bias including publication bias, consistency with other studies, precision, and directness or generalisability.
2. The impact of the evidence on a decision to treat (or deny treatment). This may depend on the utility of the reported outcomes, the quality of the evidence, the number of adverse incidents encountered, the logistics of delivery of the treatment, the cost, the effect size, and an analysis of risks and benefits.

Based on their analysis of evidence quality and the impact of the intervention, Novak et al. proposed a simple traffic light system to indicate whether an intervention had a positive clinical value (Green for GO), doubtful value (Yellow), or little value (Red). This traffic light system is believed to assist the transfer of knowledge from the research to the clinical domain and facilitate decision-making. Under this system it is possible for an intervention to have a moderate level of certainty and still be strongly rec- ommended, because, for example, the potential benefits are thought to significantly outweigh the risks. Across the 64 interventions considered, 131 separate outcomes were noted. Only 6% of these outcomes received Green for GO (supporting 13 inter- ventions), with over 70% receiving an 'apply with care' (Yellow) recommendation. The authors noted that the overwhelming majority of outcomes concerned the body structures and functions domain of the International Classification of Functioning, Disability and Health (ICF).

Frankly, a ready conclusion from the work of this group is that the state-of-the-art med- icine in cerebral palsy is quite poor with the majority of treatments having little positive effect or not enough evidence to support them, or both. Even the treatments that received a 'Go for it' label may have moderate effect-sizes where a significant number of individuals in the treatment group do not benefit. It is worth a deeper investigation of EBM in cerebral palsy, and of the specific methods and conclusions of the authors of this influential paper.

As the authors state in their Discussion:

> Furthermore, using a high-level synthesis helicopter view means that specific intervention details about how the intervention took place, who benefitted from the intervention, and for how long the intervention was carried out for were not reported; clinicians would need to turn to the included papers to obtain this information.

EBM is making a very significant impact on the quality of clinical evidence presented in trials. EBM encourages the use of strong methodologies concerning randomised controlled trial (RCT) design, data analysis and governance, and reporting. But in an area like the treatment of cerebral palsy, there are ways in which the rigid practice and application of EBM may not serve our patients well. Let's look at why RCTs in cerebral palsy may be a limited vehicle for developing the clinical science and transforming outcomes for our patients. There are five principal reasons why advances in management of the person with cerebral palsy are checked.

1. The limited application of the results of trials, systematic reviews, and meta-analyses to the clinic (knowledge transfer)

EBM, as practised, promotes the response of the group to an intervention over the response of the individual. However, the clinician, in collaboration with the patient and the patient's parents in the clinic, must make a decision on an individual's care. How could results from trials be expressed so that they facilitate this discussion? In Chapter 2, we discussed the idea of using more explicit statistics representing the probability of the success (or failure or equivocal result) from the proposed intervention. Let's apply them here to the case of José. Four years ago, José had a significant dynamic ankle equinus (increased plantarflexion in walking compared to the resting state) that was perceived to be affecting his walking function. José and his parents visited their local paediatrician, Dr Challis, to discuss the merits of injecting botulinum toxin A (BTX-A) to José's calf muscles. Dr Challis is an unusually academic type, and he had read the Novak et al. article. He recalled that BTX-A had a Green Light for improving walking function, and recommended BTX-A to the family, who agreed. He did not read, in detail, the systematic reviews cited by Novak et al. or the RCTs cited by those reviews, but perhaps he should have done. How might the conversation with the family have developed differently?

Novak et al. based their Green Light conclusion on three systematic reviews, which in turn cited many RCTs. The highest-quality RCTs are those that compared BTX-A injections to sham saline or serum injections because the allocation to the treatment or control groups is blinded (although, even in these instances, allocation may become apparent due to the side-effects of the treatment). There were only three of these cited in the collection of systematic reviews, and we will apply the results of one of them. Among the strongest positive results, in the study conducted by Bjornson et al. (2007), were improvements in performance dimension of the Canadian Occupational Performance Measure (COPM) at 12 weeks after injection and in the GMFM-66 at 24 weeks. These are tabulated in Table 5.1.

Table 5.1 Selected significant results from Bjornson et al.

Measure	Interval	BTX-A, mean (SD)	Control, mean (SD)	p
COPM (performance)	12wks	1.7 (1.4)	1.2 (1.7)	0.04
GMFM-66	24wks	3.1 (11.2)	1.2 (11.3)	0.001

COPM, Canadian Occupational Performance Measure; GMFM-66, Gross Motor Function Measure-66; BTX-A, botulinum toxin A.

Although the statistical significance does suggest a difference between the groups in favour of BTX-A, it does not state the most important thing to a clinician and the family – what is the chance of this (my) child benefitting from the treatment? In Chapter 2, we suggested alternative statistics to *p*-values to quantify this likelihood (the odds ratio [OR] and the OR for a clinically significant benefit). It is difficult to calculate these parameters from the paper without access to the raw data due to assumptions about the distribution of the data. However, we can estimate these statistics by performing Monte Carlo simulations of the data (based on the mean differences and standard deviations in COPM and GMFM-66 from Table 5.1 and an assumption of normality). We did this in MS Excel. You should try it if you have a nerdy tendency or a nerdy colleague. In the simulation, we calculated an OR of around 1.3 for GMFM-66 and 2.6 for the COPM, which means that the odds are about 4 to 3 (or 5 to 2 for the COPM) that José would benefit from the injections more than he would benefit by not having them. This seems far from conclusive. The arithmetic becomes even less persuasive if his chances of benefitting by a meaningful difference are calculated. Minimum clinically important differences of between 2 and 4 points have been estimated for the GMFM-66 and between 1.5 and 3 points for the COPM. If we adopt the lower, more conservative value, then the ORs for a clinically significant benefit are about 1.1 and 1.3 respectively. (These results represent the mean result of many repeat simulations. The variation in the simulation results suggest that it is difficult to estimate ORs with precision from studies the size of Bjornson et al.'s.) In other words, the chances of benefiting from BTX-A injections over doing nothing at all are quite small. With results expressed in this way, rather than by *p*-values, and noting that many of the other outcome measures did not reach significance, Dr Challis and the family may have moderated their expectations from treatment, and even decided not to go ahead.

It's not all bad! Some of the RCTs indirectly cited by Novak and colleagues produced reasonable effect sizes. Constraint-induced movement therapy (CIMT) for improvement received a strong Green Light. CIMT is a technique in which the non-affected (or less-affected) upper limb is constrained in a cast. The theory goes that the child is forced to use the paretic limb, developing skills in the use of that limb that they hitherto did not possess. There are modified forms of CIMT and sometimes CIMT is combined with a dose of bimanual therapy. The mechanisms behind the intervention are somewhat unclear though many believe that neuroplastic changes take place in the CNS secondary to altered use. We 'simulated' the data from one of the contributing RCTs to this positive judgement in order to calculate ORs and ORs for a clinically significant benefit. Aarts et al. combined a CIMT (6 weeks) with a shorter period of bimanual training (2 weeks) (Aarts et al. 2010). One of their reported primary outcome measures was the Assisting Hand Assessment (AHA) (Krumlinde-Sundholm et al. 2007). The other primary measure was the ABILHAND for which we could find no data on minimal clinically important differences (Arnould et al. 2004). Their significant results shortly after intervention are summarised in Table 5.2.

We again calculated the OR and the OR for clinically significant benefit (AHA only) assuming the data for the primary outcome parameter is normally distributed. The OR for the AHA was around 2, meaning that the individual child with unilateral cerebral palsy would have twice the chance of benefitting from CIMT as from standard care. When we apply the minimal clinically important difference then, around 60% of participants would

Table 5.2   Change in the mean scores (SD) on the Assisting Hand Assessment (AHA) performance measure and on the ABILHANDS questionnaire (Klingels et al. 2010)

Measure	Interval	CIMT, mean (SD)	Usual care, mean (SD)
AHA	1 week	6.8 (8.2)	2.5 (6.3)
ABILHANDS	1 week	7.5 (4)	1.1 (4.8)

CIMT, constraint-induced movement therapy.

have benefitted from constraint as opposed to 32% on usual care. Interestingly, less than 10% of children would have suffered a loss in bimanual function after CIMT against 12% receiving usual care. In this instance, the consulting clinician may advise the family of the benefit of CIMT with some security, acknowledging that the study was not blinded with all the intrinsic biases that that may confer (see Chapter 2).

These examples are simply meant to be illustrative of the way data could be presented in papers to better inform the decision-making of clinicians and families. Indeed, OR or the modified version we represent here, may not be the most statistically acceptable methods of computing a clinically meaningful effect size (Kraemer and Kupfer 2006), largely because they are binary representations of the clinical effect of the treatment and control (better or worse), and do not map easily onto other measures of effect size such as numbers needed to treat or success rate difference. Nevertheless, these simple measures are easily understood by the practitioner. Unfortunately, the effect sizes reported in the RCTs cited indirectly in Novak et al.'s review are rarely in a form readily interpretable by the reader who wishes to know the probability of their individual patient benefiting by a clinically significant amount from the treatment investigated.

Even if ORs were calculated in these papers, the study sample sizes in RCTs in cerebral palsy tend to be very small. For example, in the RCTs cited by a recent Cochrane review on botulinum toxin on spasticity management, the median sample size was 40. Precise estimates of derived parameters (OR, etc.) and their confidence intervals require precise estimates of the mean treatment effect and the variation in response to treatment. The estimate of the expected treatment effect improves with sample size, so it may be that many of these more meaningful parameters may not be estimated reliably.

Small sample sizes lead to at least two other significant problems in the conclusions drawn from RCTs, which affect knowledge transfer to the clinic.

a. Unfortunately, RCTs in cerebral palsy are rarely powered to adequately assess these possible interactions between patient factors (examples: age, sex, level of mobility, etc.) and the treatment being evaluated. Subgroup analyses are important because it is possible that the effect of the treatment in a group of patients with a particular characteristic may be beneficial, while treatment in the absence of that characteristic may not be beneficial or have a negative effect on outcome. This kind of personalisation is very difficult to do in research practice because of the potential sample sizes involved. If we decided to fully account for the factors listed above using stratification (then we might need four age groups, two sexes, and five levels of mobility) and our sample size calculation suggested that we need at least 24 participants in each stratum, then we would need 960 participants in our trial!

b. A further issue is that combinations of treatments may have a greater impact than individual treatments. In other words, the interactions of treatments may have a disproportionate effect on outcome versus the isolated effect of an individual treatment. While this is, in principle, testable by an RCT, the sample size required to assess the performance of individual treatments and the combination of treatments would be inflated.

2. The statement of the original hypotheses and the poor correspondence between hypotheses and outcome measures

RCTs were developed to reduce the biases associated with observational or longitudinal non-randomised experimental studies. Many potential biases that persist in RCTs in the area of physical medicine have already been explored in Chapter 2 including the lack of blinding of assessors and patients, comparison with placebo controls, reporting biases, etc. One issue that we have not yet discussed is Hypothesising After the Results are Known (HARKing). This is the practice of selecting a positive result from the data produced by a clinical trial or experimental study and stating falsely that this was the a priori or original hypothesis of the authors (Kerr 1998). The formation of a hypothesis may be an anathema to some. HARKing is so embedded in the minds of clinical researchers that it may not be viewed as cheating. When the authors of this book submitted their first paper in the area of cerebral palsy, one of the reviewers could not accept the results of the work because they conflicted with the hypotheses that we had made. HARKing is prevalent in clinical research, and it is extremely hard to detect. Fortunately, it is relatively easy to avoid. The researchers can employ the offices of an independent data governance committee to which the original design and hypotheses are submitted or they can register their research in advance on a centrally-held database. Alternatively, the authors can publish the design of the study and the hypotheses in advance of conducting the trial.

p-hacking is a related phenomenon in which many tests of significance are conducted with the implication that many original hypotheses have been made (Head et al. 2015). Researchers may then deselect statistical tests that did not reach significance and report only those that are positive. HARKing and p-hacking are likely to occur when researchers have not properly examined the evidence to date (i.e. previous trials, observational or experimental studies, or cellular or physiological science), and, therefore, are not in a position to make informed speculations (hypotheses). In many RCTs, including the excellent ones conducted by Bjornson et al. (2007) and Aarts et al. (2010), many more implicit hypotheses are made (many more statistical tests are conducted) than original hypotheses were stated.

This approach leads to controlled trials being constituted without adequate scientific reasoning using either outcome measures that are not directly related to the hypotheses or multiple outcomes measures that are used to address a single hypothesis. In a well-constructed trial, a single hypothesis should be paired with a single outcome measure. You may think that these arguments are a little arcane but imagine Dr Challis had dived deeper into the literature and read the RCTs. He may have been drawn to the 'significant' results rather than allow for the fact that the authors had decided to make multiple implicit hypotheses by creating multiple statistical tests.

Harking and *p*-hacking are certainly prevalent in the scientific community but there is also a danger of making too many hypotheses and corresponding statistical tests. A multiplicity of hypotheses may lead to type II errors (that is, the data analysis fails to detect one or more hypotheses which are true) where statistical tests are appropriately corrected but where many of the implicit hypotheses are not properly founded in an understanding of the science.

3. The evaluation of treatments instead of treatment approaches

As we have seen in Chapter 2, groups are made up of individuals, who, because of their differing intrinsic characteristics and environments may respond very differently to intervention. There certainly is a tension in clinical trials between recruiting a large enough sample, to adequately power a study, and having a group of participants whose presentations are similar enough to expect a narrow range of responses. Typically, clinical trials compare specific interventions with others or with a control, but there is a case, in a heterogenous population, to compare treatment philosophies. This approach would mirror clinical practice. An RCT might compare stretch-casting to usual care in the management of a child with an equinus gait and mild plantarflexion deformities, but it is rare that clinical units would limit themselves to a single intervention.

José is being reviewed by his orthopaedic surgeon, Denise Bellancourt. She is considering recommending serial casting to correct his plantarflexion deformities. Jen, José's erstwhile physiotherapist, is also attending. Jen is a part of a team that is completing a Cochrane review in serial casting. Jen has read Novak et al.'s review of reviews, which indicates that serial casting should have a Green for 'Go for it' label. The clinicians agree that although José has the level of deformity that may be corrected by serial casting, they are worried by the recent development of mild deformities at more proximal levels, and by José's mild valgus foot posture. Denise and Jen are discussing treatment options with the family. They acknowledge to José's parents that best current evidence points to using serial casting but express their concerns about the possible future progression of José's proximal and foot deformities. The family respond positively to explanations offered by Jen and Denise, and add that José did not respond well to serial casting when it was tried previously at another centre. Together, they agree to take a surgical route with lengthening of the hamstrings, calcaneal osteotomies of the feet, as well as gastrocnemius recessions. The clinicians are using their knowledge of José, of the structure of their own local services, and an internalised algorithm which accommodates José's physical presentation including the recent development of deformities, in order to obtain (they believe) the best clinical outcome. Are they wrong? In fact, they are practising EBM as Sackett and others envisaged, acknowledging the scientific literature (with its support for serial casting in the lower limb) while using their experience to make a judgment in the context of the individual in front of them.

Could we incorporate the experience and rationale of clinicians like Denise and Jen into a prospective study, as well as the views of the family? An internalised understanding of a problem is difficult to accommodate within the structure of an RCT, but if competing clinical philosophies could be made more explicit, say, in the form of a *shared decision-making* model, then they could be compared even if such research would carry additional design and governance challenges.

One example of a shared decision-making model is that proposed by Reedman et al. (the ParticiPAte trial) (Reedman et al. 2017). Here, the investigators use a well-founded theoretical approach (self-determination theory) (Deci and Ryan 2000) to gather knowledge of the child's impairments, their environments, and the views of the child, their parents, and siblings to inform goal-orientated motivational interviews in order to increased physical activity as measured by the COPM and actigraphy. They intend to compare this structured individualised-approach to standard care in a waiting-list design. Similar designs could be adapted to assess alternative impairment-focused interventions, such as serial casting botulinum toxin injection or orthopaedic surgery.

In Novak et al.'s review, trials of this nature were excluded from analysis. It is rather illogical that in an area of medicine where the impacts of even the best treatments are moderate and variable, we think of the comparative RCT of a single intervention as the best way to provide evidence to inform clinical practice.

4. The lack of research studies that incorporate outcome measures at the level of the pathology

In our vignette, José's aunt Maria was concerned that so little was known about biological basis for the impairments observed in cerebral palsy. She comes from a cancer research lab where discovering the mechanism for a disease process is of central importance to the development of effective treatments. In her world, there is not much interest in clinical studies. Instead, she is interested in how certain genes that promote cell mitosis overexpress themselves, and how their action might be moderated by a greater understanding of non-coding RNAs, and their control through epigenetic drugs (Wang 2018). She performs highly controlled laboratory experiments on cells to elaborate fundamental mechanisms. Her recent published work is thought to represent a significant step in the potential treatment of many cancers. Historically, cell and molecular research, which have elaborated cellular mechanisms in cancers and other diseases, have led to treatments that have improved survival rates dramatically.

RCTs are an important methodology in demonstrating a statistical correlation between a putative cause and effect, but that is only a part of what is required to advance the science and elaborate the causal relationships. Understanding mechanism is required to develop a model of the disease process and how to continue to treat it more and more effectively. The requirement for a pluralism of evidence to support conclusions about causation from clinical research was stated eloquently by Austin Bradford Hill, one of the most important figures in the history of medical statistics, a coauthor on the world's first successful RCT (*BMJ* 1948), and commonly perceived to be the architect of the modern RCT. In a lecture given to a section of the Royal Society of Medicine in 1965, he gave nine different considerations in the assessment of causality (Hill 2005). These are summarised and elaborated in the context of cerebral palsy in the passages below.

1. *Strength of association.* In terms of interventions, this is the difference in response in the treatment arm and the control arm. Say, a new treatment aimed at improving ambulatory mobility in cerebral palsy produces an increase in step count among participants in a research study of 4 times that of the control, then that would strongly support

the argument that the intervention and outcome were causally-linked. However, if the intervention produced only a 5% improvement in step count, we may be more sceptical of the causal link, considering any bias in the study, sample size, and random effects. Equally, a weak association does not necessarily imply a non-causal relationship, it may simply imply a moderate degree of efficacy.

2. *Consistency between studies.* This refers to evaluation of the intervention under different circumstances (different researchers, different environments, different times), and is a very important concept in establishing the external validity of a research hypothesis. External validity refers to the applicability of the results from the study population to the greater population that the intervention is aimed at (the target population). Our outcome measure of step count may have been influenced by the demographic of the study population (urban vs rural setting, socio-demographic status, average level of disability, age, sex), the quality of the research groups, and the timing of the intervention (did it take place during the winter/summer, during a disease outbreak, etc.). If this study had been repeatedly performed under a variety of circumstances, and the results were all positive, then we could have some assurance that the intervention is applicable to the patient sitting in front of us. It is a concern that different committees and groups who reflect on the evidence to support an intervention consider a *single* well-conducted RCT as high level evidence.

3. *Specificity of the intervention.* This condition may not always be required to support the causal relationship between treatment and outcome, but it is an important consideration. Let's provide an example. Single-event multilevel surgery is a treatment philosophy in which multiple procedures are performed on the individual patient with cerebral palsy with the aim of improving the gait or other aspect of function with a single intervention. Although the clinical reasons to perform these procedures are clear (e.g. children with cerebral palsy often have deformities at the hip, knee, and ankle), establishing the link between cause and effect of the component procedures is difficult when the individual surgeries (e.g. hamstring lengthening) may have effects at multiple joint levels.

4. *Temporality.* This factor may be important when we are considering alternative possible causes for an effect from an intervention. Dynamic equinus is one of the most common features of the child with spastic cerebral palsy (Wren, Rethlefsen, and Kay 2005). Botulinum toxin is proven to reduce dynamic equinus (Eames et al. 1999). But how? Botulinum toxin blocks the release of acetylcholine from nerve ending into the neuromuscular junction. The reduction in activation of the calf musculature may, in itself, result in improvement in the ankle position but its direct effect may only last a few weeks. Yet, reduction in ankle equinus may persist for many months or longer. There is a debate in the literature concerning the atrophic effects of botulinum toxin. It is possible that the longer-term effects are due to atrophy of the calf muscles secondary to a profound lack of muscle activation. Understanding precisely the temporal relationship between putative causes (loss of activation or atrophy) and their effect (reduction in ankle equinus) could be salient to deciding whether the individual patient benefits from injection or not.

5. *Biological gradient or dose–response relationship.* Hill and his colleague Richard Doll were fascinated by the relationship between cigarette smoking and lung cancer. In their observational studies they found a linear relationship between the daily number of cigarettes that smokers reported that they had smoked during their lifetime and their

chances of having lung cancer. It is unsurprising that exposure to a carcinogen and the incidence of disease are highly related. The dose–response curve may sometimes be less linear! Nevertheless, we should be able to predict the response of the individual from the magnitude of the intervention. For example, injection of a greater concentration of BTX-A should reduce muscle activation by a greater degree. If it did not, one might doubt the nature of its action.

6. *Plausibility*. Ideally, to support a causal claim, we should have a biological (or other) explanation of the statistical association between cause and effect, but knowledge of the relating mechanisms may not always be available at the time. Lack of mechanistic justification should not prevent a treatment with evident utility from being recommended. However, seeking an explanation of how an intervention has worked may be useful in two ways. Explanatory validity is an important concept for advancing and directing the scientific conversation particularly in an area of complexity where knowledge of mechanism is lacking. For example, in a study of a new strengthening programme, it may not be adequate scientifically to record the changes in voluntary strength of the participants. One should also include measurements that inform us of *how* a change was achieved. At the level of the tissue, did the participants in the study increase their myofibrillar content; was there a reduction in the fat and connective tissue in the targeted muscles; was cocontraction of agonist-antagonist muscle pairs reduced? At the level of the muscle cell, was mitochondrial function improved, were the lengths of the sarcomeres normalised? At the level of the cell, were certain genes upregulated or downregulated? Were any of these alterations at the level of the tissue, cellular and molecular levels associated with increases in voluntary strength and improved mobility? Subsequent research could then develop their programmes to emphasise one or two elements that were successful and concentrate on alternative strategies to improve the others.

7. *Coherence*. This refers to consistency between different types of data sources. For example, one might consider inconsistencies between clinical outcome data and histopathological data as undermining a proposed causal relationship. Explanation of the mechanism for the effect of the treatment protects research from some of the biases that might be present in conventional clinically-based RCTs. For example, if genes promoting increased muscle metabolism were upregulated by the intervention and correlated with improvement at the level of structure and function, and if certain other genes were not affected, then this might point to biological mechanisms depressing the rate of muscle growth in this population. Variation in treatment response may well be explained by variation in the biology of the individual or the interaction of their biology with the intervention, which would potentially mean that the application of the treatment could be *personalised.* If any improvements in strength were not associated with changes in the morphology, or physiology of the muscle or central nervous system, then we could question the validity of the trial (were the participants acclimatised to the test or were their levels of motivation to do the testing increased by participating in a rigorous training programme?).

8. *Experiment*. Hill wrote down his considerations for causality long before the emergence of EBM. Here, he recognises the potential power of controlled experiments, such as RCTs, over that of observation. He suggested that experimental results are the single strongest support for causation.

9. *Analogy.* If causality was established in one intervention, it is sensible to propose that a different, but similar, intervention would behave similarly. For example, we might expect that if causality was proven for serial casting i.e. that it consistently improved ankle dorsiflexion, then we might surmise that any procedure that held the ankle in a similarly dorsiflexed position for a prolonged length of time (say, by an orthosis) might result in a similar outcome.

Russo and Williamson pointed out that Hill's guidelines fall broadly into two groups: those that are concerned with how cause and effect are related by mechanism (3, 4, 6, 7, and 9) – they are essentially disease/intervention specific concerns – and those that are concerned with size of difference or similarity (1, 2, 5, and 8) – essentially numerical constructs that are independent of the disease under study (Russo and Williamson 2007). It may not be necessary to successfully work through all of Hill's guidelines to convince oneself of a causal relationship between intervention and outcome, but it is probably worth giving each one some consideration before reaching any conclusion about your scientific claims.

In short, RCTs may inform us if a treatment works on average, but they may not tell us how it works. Research into the mechanisms of disease and treatment may ultimately show how a treatment results in better outcomes. Cerebral palsy is a complex condition with multiple interactions between systems that are in themselves developing (see Chapter 4). Currently, the architects of clinical trials in cerebral palsy rarely recognise the complexity of the systems that they are dealing with, resulting in the slow development of our understanding the disease model, and ultimately poor progress towards better treatments.

The ideal clinical research work should include a detailed explanation of the pathologies to be treated and of the proposed effects of the intervention at the level of the pathology. In addition, outcome measures that are directly related to the explanatory model of the pathology should be included. Here, we are not talking about the 'impairments' that we would place under the body structures and functions banner in the ICF but rather biological markers that are central to our understanding of the disease process.

In the case of José's visits to Dr Challis or Dr Bellancourt, knowledge of the effect of botulinum toxin, surgery, or serial casting at the level of the cell coupled with José's own physiological and biological profile may have resulted in specific treatment regime targeted at José's particular needs.

5. Acknowledging the development of individuals with cerebral palsy across the lifespan

In the vignette at the beginning of this chapter, José's father worried about José's future development. He was right to do so. Many of the interventions that show short-term promise in RCTs show minimal positive effects in long-term follow-up studies (Tedroff et al. 2009; Tedroff, Hägglund, and Miller 2020). This is in the context of a widely-reported early decline in function in adulthood in cerebral palsy (Strauss et al. 2004).

Cerebral palsy is thought of as a neurological problem because the primary injury occurs in the brain, but recently we have become aware that the rate of muscle growth throughout childhood may have very significant consequences for long-term ambulatory mobility (Herskind et al. 2016; Noble et al. 2017). Since one of the main concerns of individual children with cerebral palsy is the maintenance of mobility, we should be circumspect

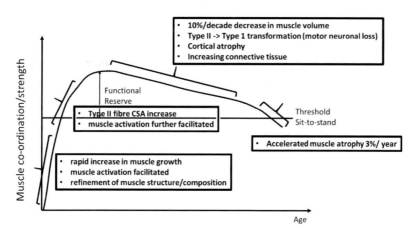

Figure 5.1 Muscular strength and control across the lifespan of the typically developing person with reference to the capacity to perform a functional task. CSA, cross-sectional area.

about the potential longer-term negative implications of short-term intervention for muscle growth. Shortland developed a conceptual model for understanding the mobility of an individual with cerebral palsy across the lifespan (Shortland 2009). In the following paragraphs, we develop this model a little further.

Figure 5.1 describes the expected development of lower limb muscle strength and control (relative to bodyweight) across the lifespan for a typically developing person. During the first year of development, there is a rapid increase in muscle growth funded, in part, by the differentiation and merging of satellite cells (the stem cells of the muscle) to form the myoblasts (muscle cell precursors), in part by the refinement of connective tissue which directs and integrates muscular effort, and by the facilitation of muscle activation through the lowering of the thresholds of alpha motor neuron activation and the promotion of activity-dependent growth (Clowry 2007). These early transformations in muscle size, structure, activation, and control allow us to pass certain motor milestones during our development, including 'sit-to-stand'. Early in childhood, we develop more muscle cross-sectional area allowing us to exceed the threshold for performing the task and develop a functional reserve, until we reach an optimum in the relationship between our muscle strength and control, and our bodyweight (Webber and Barr 2012). At this point, we could say that we have developed our maximal functional reserve. In practice, this means we have easily enough muscular capacity to achieve the task of sitting-to-stand, and indeed could probably complete the task without much trouble many times before we became fatigued. Unfortunately, from our third decade there is a slow decline in muscle strength as we lose some muscle fibres and some motor neurons, and as the quotient of connective tissues in our muscles increase (McCormick and Vasilaki 2018). Perhaps, this steady decline from our 20s to our 50s is not so noticeable in pursuing the activities of daily living but would be felt more keenly were we asked to perform an athletic pursuit that required more muscle power (this would raise the threshold for achieving the task). As we approach our old age, our muscle atrophy accelerates ultimately resulting in our inability to perform activities of daily living the sit-to-stand task (Hughes, Myers, and Schenkman 1996).

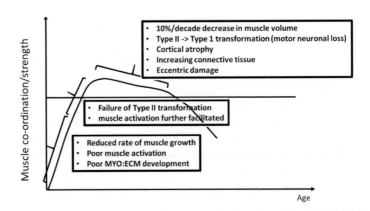

Figure 5.2 Muscle strength and control across the lifespan of the person with cerebral palsy. MYO:ECM, myofibrillar tissue to extracellular matrix ratio.

Figure 5.2 depicts how the profile of muscular strength and coordination may be altered in the individual with cerebral palsy. There is considerable evidence that the rate of muscle growth is lower in children with spastic cerebral palsy than their typically developing peers from infancy to early adulthood (Herskind et al. 2016; Noble et al. 2017). In addition, the child with spastic cerebral palsy may have difficulty activating all their muscular resources during a task (Stackhouse, Binder-Macleod, and Lee 2005), and activating them in the right order (Tedroff, Knutson, and Soderberg 2006). These factors would delay the acquisition of motor milestones such as sit-to-stand, and logically would give rise to a smaller optimal functional reserve in early adulthood than their typically developing peers. If these deficits in muscular strength are significant enough, then the child may never attain the ability to sit-to-stand. As a consequence of the diminished functional reserve and the natural history of muscle decline during adulthood, individuals with cerebral palsy who had gained mobility during childhood would lose their mobility earlier as adults. This picture is consistent with our understanding of the decline of mobility in younger and older adults with cerebral palsy. Strauss et al. documented an early loss of mobility over consecutive 15-year periods in a large group of individuals with cerebral palsy in California (Strauss et al. 2004). One of their principal findings was the loss of at least one level of mobility between the ages of 25 and 40 years in 33% of their study population.

One should consider this model when deciding on treatments for the child with cerebral palsy. According to our model, it seems that the development of an optimal functional reserve is an important factor in preserving mobility in adulthood, and it would be important to work to develop this reserve in childhood.

Equally, we should be concerned that interventions, which could compromise muscle properties in order to facilitate mobility in childhood, may give rise to a smaller *optimal functional reserve* and ultimately an earlier loss of mobility in adulthood. What little information there is in the literature suggests that some of our focal interventions do result in a level of muscular atrophy, though much more research is required to elaborate the effects of intervention on intrinsic muscle properties.

The lifespan model presented is plausible, but it is not validated. One may find it difficult to demonstrate the relationship between compromised muscle development in childhood and the loss of mobility in adulthood or the longer-term effects of intervention, by an experimental study. Instead, it may be necessary to gather evidence from observational studies over a period of decades to elucidate these relationships. Inclusion of additional measurements (e.g. muscle strength and size) in longitudinal studies similar to those by Strauss and colleagues may help us to tease out essential causal relationships between pathophysiological mechanisms, interventions, and function over the lifespan. In the case of José, we may be able to offer him and his family a more accurate prediction of his potential level of mobility in adulthood and guidance on the best way of reaching it.

SUMMARY OF THE WEAKNESSES OF EVIDENCE-BASED MEDICINE WHEN APPLIED TO CEREBRAL PALSY

Double-blinded RCTs are often the best method of proving or disproving the effectiveness of treatments particularly when applied to large-scale, well-controlled, and representative sample populations where the expected response is large. However, in cerebral palsy, these conditions are seldom met. In the preceding section we discussed in some detail the limitations of RCTs in developing knowledge and informing practice in the field of cerebral palsy. Below, we summarise our thoughts.

1. The mean response in RCTs is often moderate while the variability in response is wide resulting in effect sizes that are small, limiting translation to clinical practice.
2. The size of the sample is commonly too small to stratify the data or adjust the results according to potentially important cofactors.
3. It is difficult to double-blind treatment studies effectively (or at all) rendering the results open to significant bias.
4. Simple comparative RCTs do not capture the complex decision-making which occurs in clinical practice.
5. The follow-up period is often too short to capture long-term implications of treatment.
6. Hypotheses are often poorly developed from the existing knowledge.
7. Test statistics often do not have a stated relationship with the hypotheses.
8. There are often many more test statistics than hypotheses.
9. Outcome measures do not generally include responses to intervention at the level of tissue, cell, or molecule.
10. RCTs are difficult to perform in irreversible and significant interventions such as neurosurgery or orthopaedic surgery.

BUILDING THE EVIDENCE FOR TREATMENT: ENHANCING THE POWER OF OBSERVATIONAL STUDIES

Observational studies have been considered inferior to RCTs for well-established reasons. In principle, an RCT helps us to control for confounding variables by randomisation of all potentially influential variables (confounders) between groups except for the intervention under study, while an observational study does not control for these confounders. Yet, a review from the Cochrane Methodology Review Group suggested that observational studies produce similar effect sizes to RCTs across many different treatment modalities in spite of possible inherent biases (Anglemyer et al. 2014). As the authors conclude:

> … there is little evidence for significant effect estimate differences between observational studies and RCTs, regardless of specific observational study design, heterogeneity, or inclusion of studies of pharmacological interventions. Factors other than study design per se need to be considered when exploring reasons for a lack of agreement between results of RCTs and observational studies.

The recent availability of diagrammatic techniques and statistical tools enhance the capacity of observational studies to robustly demonstrate causal effects. One of the advantages of employing diagrammatic techniques is that they encourage you to think deeply about the possible relationships between the variables under study, and even those that you may not have included! Because potentially confounding variables are controlled in an RCT, it is possible to perform a study without reflecting too much on causal links. This is, at once, a procedural advantage and a brake on the development of the clinical science.

In the following sections, we give a brief overview of one of these tools.

A Basic Introduction to Directed Acyclic Graphs

When controlling for potential confounders in an intervention study, one needs to carefully unpick the possible relationships between the treatment, the effects of the treatment, and any likely confounding influences. Directed acyclic graphs (DAGs) are a means of displaying these relationships graphically so that assumptions behind the study design can be made explicit, and the characteristics of the participants or the environment can be adjusted for. These diagrams can inform the design of any prospective observational study (or RCT) so that appropriate statistical analyses can be carried out.

The simplest DAG consists of just two nodes and a directed arrow (Fig. 5.3).

In practice, DAGs are likely to be more complex. In the following sections, we introduce nodes in our DAG which may influence our understanding of the relationship between treatment and outcome.

Confounders

In our specific example, we might expect that there are common variables which influence both exercise and physical activity. These are termed confounders. In Figure 5.4, we introduce two of them. We might expect nutrition to influence both the physiological response to exercise of the participants and their readiness to perform physical activities. The presence of confounders or a confounder opens a *back door path* (Pearl 2010) between exercise and physical activity giving rise to a statistical association which is non-causal. In an RCT or an observational study, we could correct for this aberration by conditioning

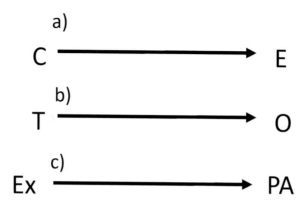

Figure 5.3 Simple directed acyclic graphs (DAGs). The figure utilises the generic language of DAGs, where C is cause and E is effect. The arrow implies a directed relationship between the two nodes, C and E, i.e. C *causes* E. When describing interventions, it is perhaps more fitting to use the term treatment (T) and outcome (O) (Fig. 5.3c). In Figure 5.3c we make the specific causal link between a treatment in cerebral palsy (physical exercise, Ex) and a measurable outcome (physical activity, PA).

on (adjusting or controlling for) *nutrition* to reveal any underlying relationship between exercise and physical activity. In the example in Figure 5.4, if the exercise intervention is randomised (say, to exercise or no exercise) then the link between *nutrition* and *exercise* is broken, the backdoor path is closed, and the direct causal relationship between *exercise* and *physical activity* evaluated.

The advantage of an RCT is realised further when the confounders are not anticipated or cannot be measured because they are likely to be evenly-distributed between the control and treatment groups, though, this cannot be guaranteed (in Fig. 5.4, the link between the *unknown* variable and exercise is broken, if the allocation to exercise/non-exercise is randomised).

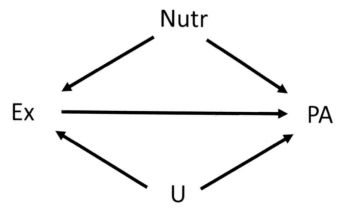

Figure 5.4 Observational studies are vulnerable to confounding if they are not anticipated or are unknown (U). Ex, physical exercise; Nutr, nutrition; PA, physical activity.

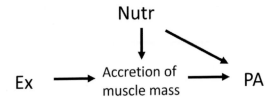

Figure 5.5 A mediator is introduced suggesting a mechanism by which exercise (Ex) influences physical activity (PA). Nutr, nutrition.

MEDIATORS

Intermediate variables or mediators can help to further elaborate our causal model by implying a mechanism between treatment and outcome. In our example DAG, we could introduce an extra node, accretion of muscle mass, in the directed path between *exercise* and *physical activity* (Fig. 5.5). Recognising a proven causal relationship between nutrition and muscle growth, we alter our DAG to include a directed path between *nutrition* and *accretion of muscle mass*. Imagine that, after adjustment of any confounders, we found that there was a weak association between *exercise* and *muscle accretion* (and therefore a weak association between *exercise* and *physical activity*) but a much stronger association between *muscle accretion* and *physical activity*. Then, we might consider methods other than exercise to increase muscle mass, such as electrical stimulation or local muscle growth factors with the aim of improving levels of physical activity.

A treatment may have multiple actions on an outcome either directly or indirectly. In a DAG, this would be represented by parallel paths in a causal diagram (Fig. 5.6) either directly, or indirectly through a mediator. In our DAG, we could include putative paths indicating a positive influence of exercise on psychological wellbeing, which in turn positively influences physical activity. In planning a study (either an RCT or an observational study), we would then incorporate a measure of wellbeing, as well as muscle size as an

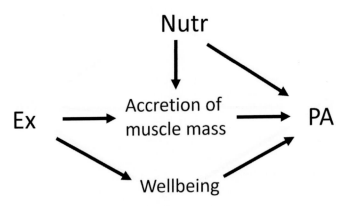

Figure 5.6 Inclusion of wellbeing as a mediator between exercise (Ex) and physical activity (PA). Nutr, nutrition.

outcome measure. Now, we have a DAG which combines biological and psychological explanations/mechanisms of the effect of strengthening exercises on outcome.

COLLIDERS

In the language of DAGs, a *collider* is a variable which is influenced by two other variables (typically, these are the causal [treatment] variable or one of the mediating variables, and the outcome variable). They are potentially problematic in study design because if they are not identified correctly, and inappropriately conditioned on, they lead to selection bias, and incorrect conclusions. In Figure 5.6, we have suggested that wellbeing is a product of a programme of strengthening exercises, which then has a causal effect on physical activity. We could have equally suggested that wellbeing influences both the quality and quantity of strengthening exercises actually performed, and the tendency to do physical activity (so it would be a confounder in our model). We could even suggest that doing strengthening exercises and physical activity influences our feelings of wellness (in this case, wellbeing becomes a collider). Depending on which is the correct causal model, conditioning on wellbeing has effects on our results and conclusions. If wellbeing was, in fact, a mediating variable and we conditioned on it (either by stratification or adjustment), then we would close the path *strengthening exercises → wellbeing → physical activity* and our analysis would reveal the relationship between *strengthening → muscle accretion → physical activity*. That would be fine, as long as that was the question we wished to ask! Otherwise, if we wanted to evaluate the effect of a *strengthening programme* on *physical activity*, through all directed paths then we would not condition on *wellbeing*. If *wellbeing* was, in fact, a confounding variable, then we would want to condition on *wellbeing* to remove any spurious association between the effects of a *strengthening programme* on *physical activity* (close the backdoor path). Imagine that we thought *wellbeing* was a confounding variable but actually it was a collider, then we introduce a selection bias by conditioning on it (i.e. we distort the relationship between *strengthening exercise* and *physical activity*). In our model, one could (superficially) justify including *wellbeing* as a mediator, confounder, or collider. For this reason, careful construction of DAGs is very important and should be informed by the best available evidence of the causal links between individual nodes. Observational studies are particularly vulnerable to collider bias, but it can occur in randomised studies as well (see the 'follow-up' example in Williams et al. 2018).

Using and Validating DAGs

DAGs may be considered a purely qualitative device to inform study design. However, because they impose restrictions (constraints) on the relationships between variables, it is possible to use statistical methods to validate them, or even refine them, by suggesting the removal of nodes or the redirection of paths in the model after collection of empirical data. Statistical packages are available online to create DAGs, supply empirical data, and assess the fit of the data to the causal diagram (Textor, Hardt, and Knüppel 2011). It is beyond the scope of this chapter to explore in-depth the methods employed to exploit a DAG or to validate it. However, a method to analyse a relatively trivial example may be explained here.

   In an imagined experiment, we inject a known number of units of botulinum toxin into a specific muscle in a group of children with cerebral palsy (X), and we plan to measure

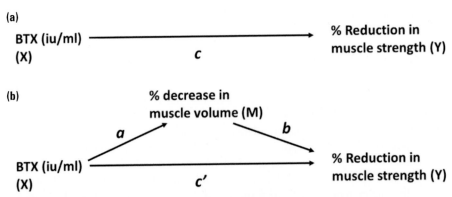

Figure 5.7 Alternative representations of cause and effect for botulinum toxin (BTX) dose in international units per unit muscle volume (X) and percentage reduction in muscle strength (Y). In model (a), effects are considered to be a direct consequence of the action of the toxin. In model (b), the effects of the toxin on muscle strength are mediated by a decrease in muscle volume (M). *a, b, c, c'* are the, as yet, unquantified, statistical strengths of the relationships between the nodes in the directed acyclic graphs.

the strength of the muscle group with dynamometry 4 weeks later (Y). We believe that the botulinum toxin will result in muscle weakness due to the action of botulinum toxin on the neuromuscular junction. Our understanding could be represented in Figure 5.7a. One plausible alternative model is that the disruption to muscle activity will result indirectly in a reduction in muscular strength secondary to muscle atrophy (M), so we decide to measure muscle volume before, and 4 weeks after, the injection. Our alternative model is represented in Figure 5.7b.

If we have measured all these variables (X, Y, and M), we are able to conduct a *mediation analysis* in which we examine the strength of each of the causal links in the DAGs in Figure 5.7, and answer the following questions:

1. Is there a causal relationship between dose of botulinum toxin (X) and reduction in muscle strength at 4 weeks post-injection (Y), and, if so, what is the strength of that relationship?
2. Is there a causal relationship between dose (X) and percentage reduction in muscle volume (M)?
3. Is the relationship between dose (X) and muscle strength (Y) completely mediated, partially mediated, or not mediated by changes in muscle volume (M)?

There are a number of ways to conduct such an analysis but perhaps the easiest method to follow is the step-wise regression proposed by Baron and Kenny (1986).

Step 1: a bivariate regression analysis is performed between X and Y. If the relationship is significant, we can estimate the strength of the relationship (*c* in Fig. 5.7a) and proceed to Step 2. If the relationship is not significant, we have no reason to proceed! From this step, we have an answer to question 1.

Step 2: a bivariate regression is performed between X and M. If the relationship is significant, we estimate the strength of the relationship (*a* in Fig. 5.7b) and we continue to Step 3. If the relationship is not significant, we would conclude that there is no *indirect* path between dose of botulinum toxin and muscle weakening due to a reduction in muscle volume. From this step we have an answer to question 2.

Step 3: a multivariate regression is performed where the explanatory (predictor) variables are X and M, and the outcome (independent) variable is Y. If the values for *b* and *c′* are significant, then the relationship between dose of botulinum toxin and reduction in muscle strength is *partially mediated* by a decrease in size of the targeted muscle. If *b* is not significant then we would say that the relationship between dose and reduction in muscle strength is not mediated by this indirect path. If *c′* is not significant but *b* is, we would argue that the effect of botulinum toxin on muscle strength at 4 weeks post-injection is *completely mediated* by reduction in muscle volume. Thus, we have an answer to question 3.

Mediation analyses, like the one outlined, help us to elaborate the theory behind the action of a medication or physical intervention by identifying causal factors that influence outcome. In the example discussed, if muscle atrophy is a partial mediator of weakness after botulinum toxin, and clinicians are concerned that atrophy-induced weakness may be only partly reversible, then they may choose to couple the injection with a dose of muscular electrical stimulation.

Improving the Evidence Base for Treatments in Cerebral Palsy by Harnessing the Power of Observational Studies

Currently, observational studies, uncontrolled trials, and other study designs occupy a low position in the hierarchy of evidence. This is due to inherent biases that can occur in non-randomised designs. As such, they are often not included in systematic reviews of the evidence or in the development of clinical guidelines. However, with the use of validated DAGs, observational and other studies may be a potent source of evidence to support or reject a treatment modality.

These sorts of studies offer some solutions to the problems we have identified with the application of the current EBM methods in conditions like cerebral palsy.

1. They permit greater numbers of participants. The sample sizes of interventional studies in cerebral palsy tend to be much larger than those in RCTs. This means that original hypotheses may be evaluated with less risk of type I or type II errors. Furthermore, effect size (such as OR) calculations for treatments may be estimated with greater precision. This would inform the conversation between clinician and family on the ratio between risk and benefit of an intervention.
2. DAGs, commonly used in epidemiological (observational) research, allow the explicit and transparent communication of hypotheses to interested scientists and clinicians. Further, they enable researchers to identify key variables to be included as outcome measures in the design of studies, including mediators that elucidate biological or

psychosocial mechanisms of cause and effect. Mandatory inclusion of DAGs in the introductory sections of research articles or grant applications could rapidly develop the science base by making transparent the thinking behind individual research works.

3. Well-conducted observational studies that include a wide range of explanatory (biological and mechanistic) variables could contribute more significantly to the evidence considered by clinical guideline committees, providing the membership of those committees included experts (basic scientists) that could verify the plausibility of mechanistic claims.

4. DAGs that have been validated by empirical studies may facilitate clinical decision-making because they help the clinician to identify factors that are pertinent to the individual patients. In this way, large observational studies may bridge the gap between EBM and patient-centred medicine. The clinician would need to answer questions posed by the following statements (see Chapter 10 in Parkkinen et al. 2018).
   • Are the crucial features of the mechanism of action in the population (the sample population in the observational study or RCT) preserved in the individual?
   • Are there further mechanisms operating in the individual that counteract the mechanism operating in the sample population?

5. Observational studies tend be of much longer duration than RCTs. In lifelong conditions, like cerebral palsy, it is essential to quantify the effects of interventions in childhood on the long-term mobility, health, and wellbeing in adulthood. In studies such as the ones conducted by Strauss et al. (2004), the inclusion of variables that might explain early loss of mobility would allow us to have a more critical view of interventions that we conduct in childhood.

SUMMARY

In this chapter, we have discussed the limitations of EBM when applied to interventions in cerebral palsy. Briefly, these include small samples sizes, moderate effect sizes, lack of long-term follow-up, and lack of personalisation of treatment. We have proposed that longitudinal non-randomised studies be weighted more heavily in the assessment of the evidence especially when the results of those studies can be fitted to a comprehensive causal model that can be justified on the basis of the existing science base and validated empirically. We believe that such research would improve knowledge transfer from research to bedside by assisting the clinician in deciding on best treatment considering the weightings of any confounding or mediating factors present in the individual.

What Does All This Mean?

Having made it this far in the book you may well have some concerns about where all this is leading. In the preceding chapters, we talked about the ways in which we agree on what we consider to be knowledge and about how we form conceptual models of reality. We talked about how we have developed ways to investigate these models of reality, and about how these models can be effective but have inherent limitations because as models they cannot by definition include all of the complexity present in reality. We have talked about potential sources of bias in research, and have discussed the limitations of the evidence available to guide our clinical management in an individual case. We have seen that our musculoskeletal system, and indeed our bodies, are not collections of independent parts; they are instead complex adaptive systems with the capacity for self-organisation, whose interaction results in emergent properties such as movement, function, and growth. These concepts are exciting and open up a range of opportunities; these include an increased understanding of what may be happening to the musculoskeletal system in children with cerebral palsy and an increased awareness of how we might use the potential for interaction of the musculoskeletal and neurological systems to enhance musculoskeletal growth and function. These concepts also, however, raise concerns about the validity of our knowledge and of our evidence base, and may appear to replace current certainties with uncertainty.

It can appear to the reader that there are only two practical responses to this uncertainty, namely a view that the musculoskeletal system in children with cerebral palsy is too complex and we do not understand it enough as yet to consider intervention, or a view that it is being presented as unnecessarily complex and we should keep doing what we are doing as we believe that it works. Neither option seems attractive as we have a continuing responsibility to provide and support optimal clinical management of children with cerebral palsy. It seems less than ideal to continue with management that may be suboptimal but equally we cannot simply decline to provide clinical care and wait for an indefinite period while our understanding of the complexity of musculoskeletal function and development increases. We need an approach that accepts uncertainty, which encompasses the complexity and nonlinearity of biological systems and the associated implications for our understanding of a clinical situation, and in this way helps guide our clinical management of the child with cerebral palsy. We can then look in this light at our clinical knowledge, and consider how we may use our understanding to develop an understanding of the balance between the risks and benefits of a particular intervention which we can discuss with the child and family and with other clinical colleagues. This is easier than it sounds!

LOOKING AGAIN AT HOW WE VIEW CLINICAL KNOWLEDGE

In the first chapter, we discussed the concept of knowledge and how it develops. In Chapter 3, we looked at how movement was not in itself predictable from consideration of the individual properties of components of the musculoskeletal system such as muscles, bones, the peripheral nervous system, and the central nervous system, which are systems in themselves. Movement could instead be considered as an emergent process arising from the interaction of these systems. In the same way, we could consider function as an emergent property arising from the interaction between the child and their environment, and could consider participation as an emergent property resulting from the interaction between the child, their environment, and society. These concepts form the basis of the International Classification of Functioning, Disability and Health (ICF), although they may not have been explicitly presented as being the outcomes of interactions between systems.

Using the same analogy, clinical knowledge could be considered not as static and objective but as an emergent property which arises from the interaction between explicit knowledge, or knowledge as defined by the clinical society, and the tacit knowledge of clinicians, which has been defined (Chugh 2015) as skills, ideas, and experiences that may be difficult to access because they may not be formally codified and may thus not necessarily be easily expressed. The tacit knowledge of a clinician will be influenced by experience; as we discussed in Chapter 1, this tacit knowledge will influence how the clinician interprets and interacts with the knowledge made explicit by the clinical society of which the clinician is a part. We discussed also in Chapter 1 the three stages involved in defining knowledge within a society as suggested by Berger and Luckmann (1966). The first stage is externalisation, where there is an agreement within a group or society regarding what is considered as knowledge. This agreed knowledge is then objectified or considered to exist independently of the individuals who contributed to its formation. The next stage is internalisation, where this knowledge is passed on to individuals entering the society and is accepted by them as objective knowledge which exists independently of the members of the society. If we consider clinical knowledge as the outcome of interaction between the clinician, the children they see, and the clinical society of which they are a part, we can see that the clinical knowledge of an individual clinician will not be static or unchanging but instead will continually evolve and develop through the interaction of new tacit knowledge gained from experience and existing explicit knowledge, which has been constructed from what would initially have been tacit knowledge but which has become codified or made explicit through interactions within the clinical society. Clinical knowledge will also involve an awareness of what is considered known and what is considered unknown, as only through an awareness of what is considered 'known' can we become aware of what is 'unknown' and vice versa. Clinical knowledge will thus involve a tension or balance between individual clinician experience and accepted clinical practice, and between what is viewed as known and unknown in terms of clinician experience and accepted clinical practice.

This may seem initially like further complexity aimed only at making the life of a clinician more difficult but instead this approach offers a way forward. Considering knowledge as a dynamic process means that we become aware that knowledge is not a fixed, objective entity but instead can be seen as a model we use to understand and interact with what in reality is a complex situation. Such a model does not need to be complete as long as it is effective; as Box (1979) stated:

> For a model there is no need to ask the question 'Is it true?' If 'truth' is to be the 'whole truth' the answer must be 'No'. The only question of interest is 'is the model illuminating and useful?'

Discussion of models reminds us of the concept of the paradigm advanced by Kuhn (1970), which was discussed in Chapter 1. A paradigm or model is effective if it helps scientists to view a topic or problem in a way that allows further progress or development of knowledge within the paradigm. The difficulty Kuhn recognised is that scientists working within a particular paradigm do not consider other paradigms. A similar difficulty in stepping outside of the models we use was expressed by Wittgenstein (1969: 16):

> All testing, all confirmation and disconfirmation of a hypothesis takes place already within a system … The system is not so much the point of departure, as the element in which arguments have their life.

THE CYNEFIN FRAMEWORK AND KNOWLEDGE DOMAINS

What is needed is a way to look at knowledge in terms of a process which helps us have awareness of the complexity of the systems we are working with and helps us identify the best approach in a particular situation. A framework for grouping knowledge into different domains, or 'sensemaking', has been proposed by Kurtz and Snowden (2003) and is called the Cynefin framework.

The Cynefin framework (Fig. 6.1) consists of four domains into which knowledge can be ordered, and a central area for knowledge or data for which the order is unclear. The four domains are termed known, knowable, complex, and chaotic. In more recent publications by Snowden, the terms simple, complicated, complex, and chaotic have been used but the earlier terms are used here as they appear more applicable in the clinical context. Before discussing the framework, it is important to consider, as Kurtz has explained, that this is not a rigid framework in that a situation may move from one category to another and that different aspects of a situation may lie within different categories of the framework.

Rather than four independent domains, we can also view the Cynefin framework as essentially two major domains, namely the right and left sides of the framework, each of which has component domains which are interrelated (Fig. 6.2). The known and knowable domains on the right side are relevant to linear systems, while the complex and chaotic domains are relevant to nonlinear systems. Linear and nonlinear systems were discussed in Chapter 3 where we saw that biological systems are inherently nonlinear, although linearity is often assumed for convenience.

The known domain relates to a situation where the relationship between cause and effect is clear, predictable, and repeatable. Kurtz and Snowden describe an approach which

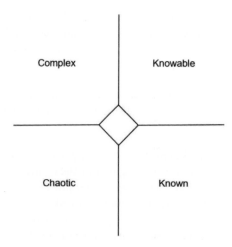

Figure 6.1   Cynefin framework.

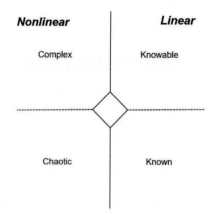

Figure 6.2   The Cynefin framework considered in terms of linear and nonlinear systems.

involves sensing (or considering) the data, categorising the data, and responding to the data (Fig. 6.3). In the known domain, best practice protocols can readily be established. The knowable domain, in contrast, involves situations where we may not immediately be aware of what is happening but where the relationships are predictable and can be understood through a process of sensing, analysing the data to define the relationships, and then responding. There may be more than one possible approach to the situation so this domain would be associated with good practice rather than a single best practice as is the case for the known domain.

The domains which involve nonlinear systems are the complex and chaotic domains. The complex domain refers to situations where we do not understand the interactions within the different components of a system; to develop an understanding we need to first

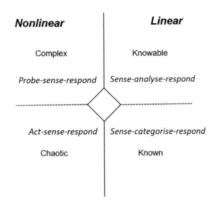

Nonlinear   *Linear*

Complex   Knowable

Probe-sense-respond   *Sense-analyse-respond*

Act-sense-respond   *Sense-categorise-respond*

Chaotic   Known

Figure 6.3   Different Cynefin domains involve different responses.

probe the system, sense the resulting changes or alterations in the system, and then con-sider how we may respond. This domain involves what is termed emergent practice, where our understanding of the system grows through interaction with the system. In the chaotic domain the interactions within the system are not predictable but are also not amenable to understanding through probing; in this situation we need to act first, then review the data. This domain is associated with novel practice.

One way of considering a complex system would be to see it as the interaction of a large number of components, each following a number of simple rules which result in complex behaviour; an example could be the movement of a flock of starlings. A flock of starlings in flight (termed a 'murmuration') can show what appears to be marked synchronisation in movement. This pattern of movement can be modelled by imposing conditions on the interaction between neighbouring birds: each bird stays at a certain distance from the other birds nearby, turns when the other birds turn, and avoids predators. These relatively simple interactions between individual birds result in the flock as a whole moving in a complex and apparently highly organised manner. A chaotic process, on the other hand, involves the interaction of a smaller number of components where a small change in the initial value of individual components leads to a different outcome which may be hard to predict accu-rately if we are not able to measure the initial values accurately. An example of this would be difficulty in predicting the weather in the UK. Chaos in this sense is not, however, random, instead it is (at least in theory) predictable nonlinearity.

In Chapter 3, we discussed the different approaches to the definitions of information and entropy, and looked at the difference between the algorithmic information content (AIC), where the complexity or information content of a string of symbols is taken to be the length of the shortest algorithm or computer program that can generate this string, and dynamical depth which looks at the different levels of organisation within a system which contribute to the overall complexity of a system. The domains of the Cynefin framework could also be derived from interaction between AIC and dynamical depth as shown in Figure 6.4, where they are shown as a continuum rather than as distinct areas within a grid.

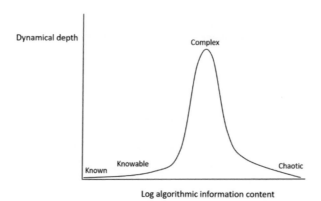

Figure 6.4 Relationship between the Cynefin framework and dynamical depth/information context (see also Fig. 3.1).

A situation where there is high regularity (low AIC) and low dynamical depth would correspond to a known domain; at the other extreme, a random system with high AIC and low dynamical depth would correspond to a chaotic domain. In between, as would be the case with most biological systems, a situation where there is high dynamical depth and moderate AIC would correspond to a complex domain. A knowable domain may arise from an assumption of linearity in a situation with low dynamical depth and mild AIC. When considering what we think we know in a clinical situation, it may first be helpful to consider which domain the situation best fits.

CLINICAL KNOWLEDGE AND THE CYNEFIN FRAMEWORK

We generally tend to consider clinical knowledge as being in the known and knowable domains. We investigate the aspects of a clinical situation that we do not know with the implicit belief that they are knowable. A randomised controlled trial (RCT) is seen as the highest level of clinical evidence, although when we consider the Cynefin domains discussed above we can see that the RCT can really only be effective for situations in the known and knowable domains, where relationships are linear and predictable. Most biological systems are nonlinear. We can apply the rationale of an RCT to a complex system, but we cannot be sure that the outcome will depend entirely on the variable we have chosen to study, as there will be interactions between the components of the system which will not be fully known or predictable. This does not mean that parametric statistical tests and RCTs are not valid; they are very effective for situations in the appropriate domain but may cause confusion or error if used in the wrong domain.

This may be why clinical knowledge, as discussed above, involves tacit and explicit components. The application or interpretation by the clinician of the explicit component of clinical knowledge in a particular situation will be influenced and informed by the tacit knowledge gained by the clinician from experience of previous clinical interactions and from the current clinical interaction. The explicit knowledge shared within a clinical society will, as noted earlier, reflect the externalisation of shared clinical experience and understanding and as a result will be likely to allow for variability both in a child's clinical presentation and in the clinician's response. Explicit clinical knowledge may not, however, be fully reliable even in a knowable situation because of the potential for bias within the clinical society in the selection of the models used in clinical practice. Explicit knowledge, and tacit knowledge, may be even less effective in a complex or chaotic clinical situation if this is viewed as a known or knowable situation. On a positive note however, we may develop an understanding of the nature of a knowledge domain through individual or shared experience, and can change our approach to a clinical situation depending on our view of the domain in which the situation can be best placed.

CLINICAL KNOWLEDGE AND UNCERTAINTY

The view of clinical knowledge as a dynamic process involving and being embodied by the clinician, rather than existing as an objective external entity, is not a new approach and has long been a part of clinical practice. When we talk about the 'art of medicine' we often refer to the first aphorism of Hippocrates (Richards 1961: 61–64):

> Life is short, and art long; the crisis fleeting; experience perilous, and decision difficult.

The term 'techne' was used by Hippocrates and is generally translated as 'art'. Techne may in one sense be taken to mean art but also means a craft, skill, or expertise. The Greek work for a healer was iatros, which comes from the Greek word 'iomai', meaning 'to heal' or 'make whole'; the same root can be seen in 'paediatrics', which could thus be translated as the craft/expertise related to the healing of children. Hippocrates used the term 'techne iatrike', which means the craft or expertise of the healer, to describe clinical knowledge. Hippocrates did not refer to an external canon of knowledge but instead to the expertise or craft of the clinician. The term 'techne iatrike' was translated into Latin as 'ars medicus', from which we get the term 'the art of medicine'. The word 'ars' in Latin, however, had a similar meaning to 'techne' in Greek, and the term 'medicus' does not refer to the academic discipline of medicine but instead to the clinician, coming from the root 'medeor', meaning to heal. The Greek and Latin terms in this way involve the concept of medicine as an embodied skill, related to the clinician, rather than an external and objective knowledge. This concept can be viewed in the context of the thought of the time. Aristotle, whose concept of knowledge was discussed in Chapter 1, was active as a philosopher after the death of Hippocrates. Aristotle used the term 'techne' to express the expertise or craft of any group or discipline; physicians and sculptors, for example, would have been viewed by Aristotle as having different but appropriate expressions of techne. He did not make a distinction between different types of techne, so for him the discussion as to whether medicine was an art or a science would not have held any meaning (of interest, the word 'science' comes from the Latin word scientia, which means knowledge, a knowing, expertness, or experience – not dissimilar in itself from the meaning of techne). 'Episteme' for Aristotle represented that aspect of knowledge which was unchanging and was part of nature, while 'techne' could be considered to represent or describe the expertise we use to deal with complex and variable events; these events were described in turn by the term 'tuche', which could be expressed as meaning 'chance' or 'fate'. Nussbaum described 'tuche' as what happened to a person, as opposed to what the person did or made; it was the element of human existence that humans do not control (Nussbaum 1986). Techne thus involved a deliberate application of human intelligence to some part of the world, yielding some control over tuche, and came into being, wrote Aristotle, 'when from many notions gained by experience a universal judgement about a group of similar things arises' (Nicomachean Ethics 98 iaj-7). This is a good description of how clinical knowledge develops. Hippocrates was aware of the potential for error implicit in clinical experience and the difficulty in making clinical decisions: 'experience perilous, and decision difficult'. He concluded his first aphorism with the following statement:

> The physician must not only be prepared to do what is right himself, but also to secure the co-operation of the patient, of the attendants and of externals. (Richards 1961: 61–64)

How are we to secure the cooperation of the child and family and to gain their confidence if we as clinicians are to acknowledge uncertainty regarding our clinical understanding and our clinical decision-making? How are we to gain the cooperation of what Hippocrates described as the externals, who may be considered as clinical colleagues, health care managers, and funding agencies, if we are not seen as knowledgeable experts? One option is to deny clinical uncertainty and hold fast to the existing clinical paradigm. Certainty seems possible if we view biological systems as linear systems of which we already have full knowledge (as in the case of a situation within the known domain) or believe full knowledge can be attained through more and larger RCTs (as in the case of a situation within the knowable domain). But biological systems are not linear; we can treat them as linear, but this is at best an approximation and as we have seen this limits our ability to look at interactions between components of the system and at interactions between individual systems and subsystems. This does not mean that we cannot have understanding and cannot be predictive to an extent regarding outcome, but it does mean that we cannot be certain about outcome or the effect of intervention on outcome. So how can we recommend intervention or proceed with intervention if we are not certain? A response, as outlined in Chapter 1, may be that the terms certainty and uncertainty are not binary concepts; rather than being either certain or uncertain there are levels of uncertainty. It is possible in theory to be 99% certain, if certainty could be quantified in this manner, but this would still mean that we are uncertain as certainty could only be held to be present if we are 100% certain.

There are different types of uncertainty. Epistemic uncertainty (from the Greek episteme, meaning knowledge) occurs when we do not have all of the information which is available; this uncertainty can be reduced in a clinical situation through training, familiarity with the published research, and experience. Aleatory uncertainty (from the Latin aleator, a dice-thrower), on the other hand, relates to outcomes which cannot be predicted such as the throw of a dice. This type of uncertainty will be inevitable to an extent when making predictions about a biological system; such a system is not random, as discussed earlier, but the outcome or trajectory of the system is sensitive to small changes in initial conditions and we do not have all of the information about the initial conditions or the interactions between the variables in the system. Aleatory uncertainty will be assumed as inherent if the clinical situation is thought to be in the complex domain. If the clinical situation is assumed to be in the known or knowable domains, uncertainty may be considered as epistemic and capable of resolution through the acquisition of more information or the verification of existing information. This may be an effective approach if this is the appropriate domain, but if we are dealing with a situation which is in a complex domain rather than a known or knowable domain, this approach will not be effective. A third type of uncertainty, ontologic uncertainty, involves situations where we do not know what we do not know. This may be because we are dealing with a new area, or because the clinical model we are using involves assumptions which exclude the possibility that aspects of the situation may not have been considered.

Acceptance of uncertainty in clinical practice would not be new, as evidenced by Hippocrates' aphorism, but in itself will not be effective in informing clinical management or in facilitating interaction with the child and family and with other clinicians. To achieve this, we will need to look more closely at how our clinical model informs our clinical approach.

A SYSTEMS APPROACH TO CLINICAL KNOWLEDGE

As discussed in Chapter 1, the current paradigm for the development of musculoskeletal deformity appears to be that muscles need to be stretched if they are to grow, and that spasticity limits this ability of the muscle to stretch, and as a consequence leads to impaired muscle growth. Our clinical model in this way involves the concept that if spasticity could somehow be reduced or removed from a muscle, the muscle would grow in a typically developing manner. This model, when considered from an external perspective, offers a relatively clear approach, and provides a clear framework for intervention, which is likely to account for its widespread acceptance. Despite (or perhaps because of) this apparent simplicity the current clinical model has limitations; it can be argued that these result from the approach we take as clinicians, in which spasticity is effectively seen as an objective or independent entity which can be managed or treated in isolation. The model involves confusion or ambiguity between our use of the concept of spasticity as an independent entity and our use of the term to mean a physical sign which can be elicited by clinical examination. There is further ambiguity in the differing current definitions of spasticity. Our current clinical model would in this way fail Box's test as it could not be considered 'illuminating or useful'.

In Chapter 3, we discussed a systems approach which allows us to consider the interactions within muscle and the interactions between muscle and other body systems which result in movement and in musculoskeletal growth. To make such a model useful in a clinical setting, it would need to be extended to include the interactions between a child's movement and the environment in which the child is developing. If we look at interactions rather than impairments, and if we consider how the outcome of the interactions between systems such as the musculoskeletal system and the nervous system allows the child to interact with their environment, then our model would have the capacity to range from the atoms of each of the child's cells to the society in which the child lives. The connection between an individual cell, or the molecules within a cell, and society is difficult to express in a linear fashion but can be considered in a nonlinear fashion if we view these interactions as a network of connections between the emergent properties of the complex adaptive systems involved.

As an example, consider a child playing a game with her friends at school. Her choice of game will be influenced by her personal preference and level of energy, and through interactions with her friends who will themselves have preferences regarding which game they would like to play. Her ability to participate in the chosen game will depend on the interactions between her musculoskeletal system and her nervous system. These interactions will also be influenced by the constraints imposed by gravity, by her understanding of the game, and by her ability to communicate with her friends. An alteration in the physical environment, in the time of day, in the preferences of the children involved or in their energy levels may result in the choice of a different game. There will be interactions and connections within each of these individual systems, some of which may not be immediately obvious. If I was to suggest a link between quantum mechanics and the child's choice of game, for instance, this could be seen as fanciful. The energy to drive movement, however, depends on the availability of adenosine triphosphate (ATP) within the muscle and nerve cells. We saw in Chapter 3 that ATP is produced predominantly through oxidative phosphorylation in the mitochondrion. This process relies on electron tunnelling by means of which an electron can traverse an apparently impenetrable barrier (Hayashi and Stuchebrukhov 2011). Without the capacity for tunnelling of electrons, there would be less ATP available, and the child's ability to play and communicate with her friends would be constrained. This is perhaps an extreme connection but will hopefully illustrate the point that our model must accept and assume interactions at all levels, some of which may be clear and some of which will not be clear.

How does our present clinical model fit into this approach? If this child had cerebral palsy, we might consider looking for a correlation between a particular impairment, such as a measure of stiffness within a muscle, which we could arbitrarily term spasticity, and the ability of a child to participate in play with her friends. As discussed in Chapter 5, we will be likely to find an association due to the interactions already present in the system, but an attempt to define a linear correlation will mask or ignore the other interactions present. If we then consider an intervention to alter what we view as an objective impairment which has a direct effect on the child's ability to play, namely her spasticity, we may be disappointed with the outcome. We could work to clarify our definition of muscle stiffness or spasticity, and the means by which we measure it, but are still unlikely to find what we can consider a causative link between an alteration in the muscle stiffness and the child's participation in the game. We need instead to see the movement, the child, and the game as an overall process involving interactions within and between multiple levels. This does not mean that we need to have a complete understanding of all levels – most clinicians (including the authors!) are not quantum physicists – but it does mean that we need to have an awareness of the network of interactions present and an awareness that intervention or alteration at one level will result in alterations, both anticipated and unanticipated, at other levels. This approach involves an awareness of movement, for example, as a process resulting from interactions between systems (between, e.g. the skeleton, muscles, nerves, and the physical environment) rather than as an objective entity which exists in itself. It is difficult, if we stop to think about it, to come up with a definition for movement which does not involve the concept of interaction.

THE ROLE OF EXTERNAL FACTORS IN SYSTEM DEVELOPMENT

We have not so far discussed the role of factors or influences external to the child, apart from availability of energy substrate in muscle development. Each of us, however, is effectively embedded or nested in other systems which interact with each other. We are each part of the physical environment and are subject to the effects of gravity and electromagnetism, as well as to the laws of thermodynamics mentioned earlier. We are also situated within a social context in which we interact with other people. As an individual, each of us can generate movement but the degree to which this movement is functional will depend on the interaction between us and our environment and will be influenced also by the social context in which the movement is performed.

We are familiar with this concept when we think about communication. Communication and language do not have a meaning independent from our social environment and involve interaction between the physical and social environments in which we exist as complex adaptive systems. Speech involves encoding a concept in sound and then producing that sound by means of forming vibrations in the air by using the vocal cords. Hearing involves decoding of these vibrations through analysis of frequency and rhythm with subsequent reconstruction of the concept expressed. Communication thus involves interaction between at least two people within a shared physical, social, and linguistic environment.

If we wanted to look at development of movement and function in a child, we could consider a state space with three axes, namely biological, physical, and social (Fig. 6.5). Each axis could reflect the outcome of a particular pattern of interactions. The physical axis could represent the interaction of the child with the physical environment, and would include movement and function. The social axis could represent the interaction of the child with their peers, with their parents, and with other adults and children, and could include communication. The biological axis could include interactions leading to growth and development of the child as a complex adaptive system. These axes are not exclusive

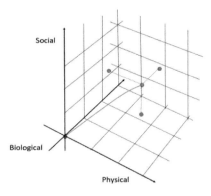

Figure 6.5 A possible state space for child development.

and will in themselves interact. Communication, as we have noted above, will involve interaction of all three axes, as will play. The interaction of these axes thus provides us with a simplified three-dimensional space within which we can consider the overall development of a child. (Of note, only three axes have been selected for clarity and for the purposes of discussion. In a complex system there are unlikely to be only three axes and these axes are unlikely to be so conveniently orthogonal!)

Progression along each axis can be represented by a single point in the three-dimensional space; this point will have been attained by following a particular trajectory in the space. Unless we have been able to follow the child's progress closely, it will be difficult for us to specify accurately the trajectory followed in reaching any point. This means that a particular point may have been reached by a number of possible trajectories, or indeed that the same point in this state space may be reached by two children on different trajectories.

IS THIS HELPFUL FOR CLINICAL PRACTICE?

The causal loop diagrams discussed in Chapter 4 are simple models for the purposes of illustration and discussion but may provide some insight into the potential effects of intervention to a complex system. We have seen that muscle growth is an energy-intensive process involving an interplay between energy availability, the state of muscle development, and the demands imposed on muscle. We can appreciate that a focus on impairment may not be helpful; the degree of stiffness or resistance to stretch of a muscle, for instance, will depend on the interaction between muscle innervation, muscle length, and the balance between contractile and non-contractile tissue and will reflect an altered trajectory of development of the muscle. The concept that removal or reduction of an impairment will result in a typical pattern of growth is difficult to support when we consider skeletal muscle as a complex system. As we discussed when considering developmental trajectories of the musculoskeletal system in Chapter 4, there is no evidence to show that we can positively alter the trajectory of musculoskeletal development and function in a child with cerebral palsy outside of its likely pre-existing range of potential outcomes. This means that a 'normative' approach, where the child is compared to a putative 'normal' child and where the goal of intervention is to provide 'normality' is not only unlikely to be effective but also fails to consider the complexities of musculoskeletal development and the limitations of our current therapeutic approach. We can see also that any intervention needs to be considered in a context which includes the child's physical and social environment.

Discussion with parents, children, and other clinicians about the complexity of the systems and interactions involved, about our difficulty in predicting or altering developmental outcomes, and hence about our difficulty in predicting future function and the impact of intervention may initially seem more likely to reduce their cooperation and confidence rather than to secure it as recommended by Hippocrates. Such an approach, however, gives us the opportunity as clinicians to review what we consider as 'facts', to consider which of these facts we consider as relevant, and to consider how we apply these judgements to clinical decision-making in the context of our values. If we appreciate the complexity of biological systems, and the degree of interaction within and between different systems, we can appreciate also that any interpretation we have of such a system will inevitably be a model of a complex reality rather than reality itself. This is not a criticism of the use of a model. As an analogy, we could consider a map; the degree of information provided by a map will be selective and the utility of the map will depend on which features are of interest to the user. A map that includes all of the available physical information on a 1:1 scale would be comprehensive but would not be usable; it would instead require another map at a smaller scale to make it comprehensible. Once we begin to appreciate that like a map, any clinical model has by definition to be selective and has to include some aspects of a complex system and exclude others, we can begin to appreciate that we approach a particular situation from our own 'reference frame'. We can also begin to understand that clinical colleagues, children, and parents may have different 'maps' or reference frames, which will be associated with a different set of 'facts' and which may see other aspects of the situation as important. We may not appreciate that each of us has a different map or model of reality which we shape individually; in the words of the psychologist William James (Wu 2011) 'My experience is what I agree to attend to. Only those items which I notice shape my mind'. He defined attention as 'the taking possession by the mind, in clear and vivid form, of one out of what seem several simultaneously possible objects or trains of thought … it implies withdrawal from some things in order to deal effectively with others' (Wu 2011). As a child, parent, or clinician the model we construct, or the way in which we view a situation, will be influenced by factors such as our experience and understanding, and our degree of comfort with uncertainty. An awareness of this can help us to look at a clinical situation in a wider context and to include other perspectives in clinical decision-making and goal setting in discussion with clinical colleagues and families. This approach is known as critical systems heuristics (CSH) (Ulrich 2005; Ulrich and Reynolds 2010).

CRITICAL SYSTEMS HEURISTICS

The central idea of CSH is that how we define a problem, how we manage it, and how we assess the outcome of intervention all depend on our prior judgements about the system in question. The term 'heuristics' comes from the Greek 'heurisk-ein', meaning to find or discover. CSH is aimed at helping us to critically understand how we make judgements about a system. As any interpretation or representation of a complex system will not encompass all of the system, we make decisions about what we view as relevant in terms of observations and values and what we view as not relevant. These decisions are termed 'boundary judgements'. This term is not intended as critical; instead, there is clear acceptance that any interpretation of a complex system has to involve boundary judgements if we are to work effectively with the system. These boundary judgements define what we see as 'facts' and 'values', these are described in CSH as 'claims'. The term 'claim' in CSH is used to describe all assertions or suggestions regarding a system to which we attach meaning and justifiability, including clinical decisions regarding intervention. The claims we make, which relate to what we consider as facts and values, are defined by how we make boundary judgements or, in other words, by how we select those aspects of the system that we view as important and relevant to a particular discussion and exclude other aspects that we view as not being relevant. The boundary judgements, together with the facts and values we view as relevant, form our reference frame from which we view a particular system. The reference frame is not necessarily fixed; a modification of our reference frame through a change in boundary judgements means that different facts and values may be seen as relevant in a particular situation. Once we appreciate that our judgements of fact and value depend on how we define our reference frame through boundary judgements, we have a way of looking at individual claims and reference frames to identify areas or agreement and disagreement.

Ulrich identified four basic boundary issues through which a claim can be assessed:

- Basis of motivation: where does a sense of purposefulness or value come from?
- Basis of power: who is in control of what is going on and what is needed for success?
- Basis of knowledge: what experience and expertise support the claim?
- Basis of legitimacy: where does legitimacy lie?

For each boundary issue, Ulrich considered three categories as shown in Figure 6.6.

The CSH framework is not aimed at providing a single correct answer in a given situation but instead at allowing claims to be explored by means of definition and exploration of the underlying boundary judgements involved. This can allow the merit of a claim to be discussed in a way that includes perspectives that may not have been included in the initial boundary judgements and in a way that can help the people involved to understand each other's reference systems and in this way come to a mutual agreement about intervention. CSH allows for reflective practice, where a clinician can critically assess their boundary judgements, and also provides a framework (known as emancipatory practice) where other clinicians or the family involved can enter discussion into clinical management options.

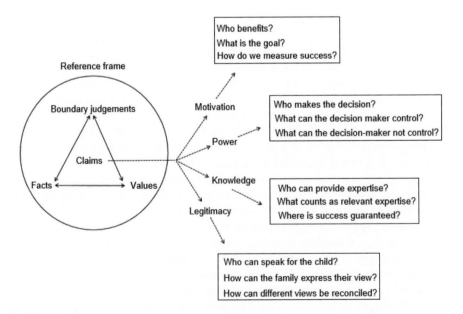

Figure 6.6 The critical systems heuristics framework.

As an example, consider a 3-year-old child with bilateral cerebral palsy, in Gross Motor Function Classification System (GMFCS) level V, referred for an orthopaedic review because of hip dysplasia. A hip radiograph done as part of a screening programme shows reduced coverage and lateral migration of the right femoral head, with a migration index (essentially the percentage of the femoral head which is not covered by the bony acetabulum) being measured as 35%. The child has severe global developmental delay, epilepsy, obstructive sleep apnoea, and feeding difficulties for which they have had a gastrostomy tube inserted. In the clinic room are the child, parents, and the orthopaedic surgeon. On examination, the child's hips are mobile and seem comfortable, and no problems with movement for activities of daily care are reported. The surgical options here would be to recommend surgical intervention or observation. Let us look first at the possible boundary judgements of the surgeon, and then at the possible boundary judgements of the parents and physiotherapist.

One approach by the surgeon could focus on the degree of migration of the hip. A migration index of 35% could be viewed as demonstrating hip dysplasia which is above a threshold index for intervention and likely to progress, with the child's GMFCS level, age, migration index, and head-shaft angle acting as relevant variables influencing the risk of progression and informing the need for early intervention (Hermanson et al. 2015). Assessment of the child's hips and a review of the radiograph may then lead to a recommendation for surgical intervention. In this scenario, the importance of the migration index would be a boundary judgement, leading to a further conclusion or 'claim' that surgical intervention should be considered. In an alternative scenario, the surgeon may again consider the migration index as a potential indication for surgical intervention, but may consider the migration index to be less relevant that the history of obstructive sleep apnoea, and may recommend that this be investigated and managed as appropriate before consideration of surgical intervention. In this scenario, the boundary judgement would relate to the risks of surgery raised by the obstructive sleep apnoea. In a third scenario, the surgeon may consider both the obstructive sleep apnoea and the migration index but may feel that ongoing monitoring rather than surgical intervention is needed because of a boundary judgement regarding the level of risk of progression of hip dysplasia associated with a particular migration index.

The child's parents will come to the consultation with different boundary judgements. The migration index in itself may be seen as relevant, depending on the discussion with the child's physiotherapist and paediatrician prior to the referral, but the child's sleep difficulties and epilepsy may be viewed by the parents as being of higher priority, particularly given the lack of any symptoms related to the hip dysplasia. The parents may see the hip dysplasia as being a limiting factor in the child's development of mobility, with the resulting hope that intervention to the hip may result in an improvement in their child's function. They may also view the process of admission for surgery with concern, as this effectively will involve handing over the care of their child to clinicians whom they feel may not know their child, and will be likely to involve pain and distress for their child who will not be in a position to understand what is happening.

Ulrich does not explicitly discuss the relevance and role of uncertainty in CSH but from our discussion earlier in this chapter we can see that both the surgeon and the parents will have areas of aleatory, epistemic, and ontologic uncertainty. For the parents, most of the uncertainty may be epistemic, which can be reduced by discussion once this is made explicit, but there will also be aspects of the uncertainty that will be ontologic in that the parents will not be aware of factors which lie outside of their experience. For the surgeon, the lack of our ability to accurately predict outcome in an individual, as was discussed in the previous chapter, may raise concern about what Lönnqvist has termed 'the number needed to suffer', which he defined as 'the suffering of other patients that is associated with one single individual having a good outcome' (Lönnqvist 2017). A boundary judgement which involves setting a lower threshold for intervention for hip dysplasia may mean that some children whose dysplasia would not have progressed will have surgery which was not needed, and which will involve pain and the risk of adverse events. Setting a higher threshold for surgery may mean that dysplasia which has progressed may need more extensive surgery than would have been the case if it was performed earlier. Allowing for this, we still do not know whether surgical intervention alters the developmental trajectory. It could be argued that for children who have had intervention for mild hip dysplasia those hips that develop recurrent dysplasia following intervention are the hips that had a marked underlying alteration of growth and development which was not altered by the intervention, and those hips which went on to develop well had a less marked alteration in their developmental trajectory and may have done well without intervention. This is an area where we find ontologic uncertainty – there are factors related to the development of hips that we do not know what we do not know.

The interaction of the surgeon and parents in terms of their individual approach to certainty is also likely to influence the outcome of the consultation. A surgeon expressing certainty regarding a recommendation for intervention is likely to be favourably received by parents who are more comfortable with certainty, and who in turn may feel less comfortable or happy with a surgeon who expresses uncertainty. Parents who are more comfortable with uncertainty, on the other hand, may be happier if involved in a consultation where the potential uncertainties around the child's treatment are discussed.

A potential concern about CSH is that everything may seem to be related to 'claims', giving an impression that all approaches and opinions are equal and that 'anything goes'. This is not the case, as the process involves a critical analysis of the evidence supporting each claim, but it can seem that the process lacks a focus. The first boundary issue discussed by Ulrich, however, includes the question 'who benefits?' suggesting that the benefit of intervention for the child should be the focus of the discussion and should guide consideration of intervention. This is not a new concept. An effective framework for the clinical management of children with cerebral palsy has been discussed by Rosenbaum and Gorter (2012) who recommended that the components of the ICF be framed as 'F-words': function, family, fitness, fun, friends, and future. Rosenbaum and Gorter distinguished function, which can be viewed as what people do, from impairments, and emphasised the importance of avoiding a normative approach where children are expected to achieve specific goals in a specific manner. Their focus on the way in which all of these components interact and on the importance of the interactions the child has with their family and friends represent an effective approach for clinicians and families, and the reader may well wonder whether we really need another model or approach. It can, however, be difficult to know how we can incorporate assessment of impairment into the approach suggested by Rosenbaum and Gorter in a way which can both be meaningful for the child and guide clinical decision-making. Clinical management of the musculoskeletal system in children with cerebral palsy frequently involves objective measures such as muscle stiffness, joint passive ranges, muscle strength, motor control, and degree of hip migration. These measures have value: surgical intervention for instance aims at altering structure with the aim of improving it and hence improving function. An objective measure may help inform the indications for surgical intervention and when repeated following surgery may be useful in assessing the outcome in terms of a change or improvement in body structure. A difficulty is that children with cerebral palsy may have a particular perspective on the interaction between themselves and their environment, which may not be encompassed by objective measures or by the ICF, as shown by the following quotations:

> I am always aware of my body as an object to be controlled, not really 'part of me', and yet – and at the same time it is certainly 'my body' which I need to constantly reorganize.
>
> (Cole et al. 2017: 1002)

> People just stare at you and they think that you are not all there, when really you are all there, it is just your legs tag along with the rest of your body.
>
> (McLaughlin 2017)

> Just don't like that arm, I just think it is flimsy and gives me away … I just think that I would want me arm chopped off and replaced with a robotic one.
>
> (Coleman-Fountain and McLaughlin 2013)

These concerns are important to the child and are valid but are difficult to relate directly to the objective measures we use and are also difficult to incorporate directly into the framework advanced by Rosenbaum and Gorter. If we are to develop a clinical approach which includes these perspectives along with the use of objective measures and the ICF we need to consider how children and young people with cerebral palsy experience themselves and the world, and to consider how to incorporate this into our clinical management approach. To consider cerebral palsy as experienced by the child, we can look at the ideas and work of two French existentialist philosophers of the 20th century, Jean-Paul Sartre and Maurice Merleau-Ponty.

SARTRE: EXISTENCE COMES BEFORE ESSENCE

The term existentialism became known publicly through a lecture given by Sartre in 1945 entitled 'Existentialism Is a Humanism', in which Sartre stated the principle that 'existence comes before essence'. To explain this principle, Sartre compared an object which is made, such as a letter-opener, with a human being. The made object needed to have already existed in thought, or 'in essence', in order for it to have been made. Sartre said that a human being, in contrast, 'exists, encounters himself, surges up in the world, and defines himself afterwards'. Sartre had previously (Being and Nothingness 1942) discussed the concepts of 'facticity', namely the body and situation that each of us has, and 'transcendence', namely how we go beyond this facticity to exist in the world as an individual 'project' (Sartre 2015).

For Sartre, there is no normative approach. Each of us is an individual project, an individual combination of facticity and transcendence, and to be what Sartre terms 'authentic' is to exist in a way which accords with this individual combination of facticity and transcendence rather than to define ourselves with respect to any objective normative goal. In the context of the clinical management of children with cerebral palsy, this concept is implicit in the framework advanced by Rosenbaum and Gorter, which avoids such a normative approach. A reading of Sartre would encourage us to see each child as an individual and particular personal process, for whom treatment goals should not be based on a normative approach but instead on the child's particular combination of facticity and transcendence.

In his book *Being and Nothingness*, Sartre discussed the ways in which we perceive ourselves. These concepts may seem complex but have relevance as we will see for the child with cerebral palsy. Sartre divided reality into inert matter, which he termed 'being-in-itself' and human consciousness, which he defined as 'being-for-itself'. Sartre described being-for-itself as an event or process which was both 'wholly body' and 'wholly consciousness', a lived or experienced body which we do not perceive as a 'thing' but instead essentially as a medium through which we perceive the word: 'The body is lived and not known'. We do not generally perceive our body but instead perceive the environment in which we are placed: 'We perceive the resistance of things. What I perceive when I want to lift this glass to my mouth is not my effort but the heaviness of the glass' (Sartre 1983: 324). Our lived or experienced body can extend outside our physical body to include a chair or a cane: 'my body always extends across the tool which it utilises: it is at the end of the cane on which I lean' (Sartre 1983: 325). A lived, experienced body (*corps-existé*) can, however, become apparent to me through illness; the descriptions of cerebral palsy above suggest that my experienced body may no longer be invisible but instead may be obtrusive.

Sartre made a distinction between my experienced body and my 'objective body' (*corps-vu*): this is my body which is measured and viewed by science and medicine. Sartre also discussed the concept of 'my body-for-others': this is how I experience my body, which I generally do not perceive, through the perception of others. In Sartre's view, I do not view my lived body as an object, and this perception of myself as an object defined through another's view may result in embarrassment or alienation. Sartre (1983: 353) wrote 'I cannot be embarrassed by my own body as I exist it. It is my body as it may exist for the other which may embarrass me', which 'becomes designated as a thing outside my subjectivity, in the midst of a world which is not mine. My body is designated as alienated'.

MERLEAU-PONTY: WE ARE ENSEMBLES OF LIVED MEANINGS

Maurice Merleau-Ponty's concept of the 'corps propre' or lived-in body, and the 'corps objectif' or objective body, was discussed briefly at the end of Chapter 1. He viewed the 'lived-in body' as both part of the world and as how we experience and define this world through our senses. He viewed the lived-in body and the objective body as intertwined, and suggested also that the body and world are intertwined. He saw a human being as experiencing and responding to the environment or world in which they are placed, and experiencing and responding to the other people in the world, through the individual's lived-in body which brings together lived experiences, the environment, and consciousness to form a coherent personal entity. Merleau-Ponty (2002: 177) wrote 'our body is not the object of an "I think": it is an ensemble of lived meanings that finds its equilibrium'.

Merleau-Ponty suggested, as did Sartre, that we are able to extend our lived-in body to encompass objects we use such as a stick so that we are implicitly aware of the stick as part of our-lived-in body, and termed this 'incorporation'. He used an example of a woman with a feather in her hat walking through a doorway while being aware of the location of the feather in relation to the doorway.

Sartre did not discuss how the lived or experienced body develops; from his writing it seems that he considered that it develops through experience, but he focused on the experience of adults. Merleau-Ponty was Professor of Child Psychology and Pedagogy at the University of Paris from 1949 to 1952 and wrote and lectured on child development. He considered children as being engaged with the world and with other people, as inherently socially interactive, and as active participants in developing a coherent interpretation of the world based on their experiences (Welsh 2013). In Merleau-Ponty's view, the child does not experience their body as an object, but experiences it as entwined with a situation in a meaningful way; there is no subjective inside nor an objective outside to the lived body (Simms 1993). The intertwining of the lived-in body and the objective body means, however, that body structure will influence how the world is perceived and constructed by the child through their lived-in body; the same environment will be perceived in different ways, for example, by a child who is independently ambulant and by a child who depends on a wheelchair for mobility. A child's interaction with their environment and their development of functional mobility will depend on the interaction between their lived-in body, their environment, and their family.

The concepts advanced by Sartre and Merleau-Ponty are echoed by current views on the child's experience of cerebral palsy. Cole et al. (2017), for example, view cerebral palsy as not only a physiological and neurological dysfunction, but also a way of experiencing the world; they discuss 'the lived world of CP [cerebral palsy] where the body, the social, and the emotional coalesce'. Sartre's approach (as discussed by Moran) and Merleau-Ponty's approach (as discussed by Mulderij) link a number of different threads of discussion throughout this chapter such as the recommendation of Rosenbaum and Gorter to avoid a normative approach in the clinical management of children with cerebral palsy, the concept of movement and function as an emergent property arising from the interaction of the child and their surroundings, and the concept of the adjacent possible where the child as a unique developing system will have particular opportunities or possibilities for further development depending on their current state and prior development (Mulderij 2000; Moran 2011).

THE CLINICAL RELEVANCE OF THE LIVED-IN BODY

In Chapter 1, we discussed how a focus on, and appreciation of, the child's 'lived-in' body in terms of how they experience their world has a number of potential benefits. It may facilitate identification and discussion of issues which are viewed as relevant and important by the child and family, may help in discussion about the goals and potential outcomes of intervention, and may emphasise the need for the clinician to consider the child as a person who is part of their world rather than focusing on an isolated impairment. An awareness of the potential adverse effect of a normative approach to intervention may help to avoid an adverse perception by the child of their body-for-others with associated embarrassment or alienation on the part of the child. This approach places the child at the centre of the discussion while maintaining an understanding of the importance of the interaction between the child's lived-in body and their physical and social environment. A focus on each child as a process involving a particular facticity (or existing biological, physical, and social situation) and transcendence (or individual capacity for development) also helps avoid a normative approach in that each child will be seen as having a particular interaction between their lived-in body and their environment, which will influence what is possible for the child in terms of mobility. This will in turn influence how we discuss treatment goals. An acceptance of the individuality of this interaction by the child, the family, and the clinicians involved may help the child to work within their adaptive possible, avoiding the equally undesirable extremes of treatment goals which underestimate or overestimate the child's potential (both of which would have been viewed as 'bad faith' by Sartre), while being supported by their family, friends, and clinicians. Locating the child in the world as a person experiencing their world through their lived-in body also provides a focus within CSH for discussion about clinical management and intervention options. These options will be informed by assessment of the child's objective body, which will remain important; the challenge will be to interpret these measures in the context of the child's lived-in body and their interaction with the world.

THE CHILD WITH SEVERE COGNITIVE IMPAIRMENT

Understanding the child's lived-in body and their interaction with the world may be a particular challenge in children with severe cognitive impairment who may not be able to communicate their lived experience. Merleau-Ponty (2002: 237) wrote 'The thing, and the world, are given to me along with the parts of my body, not by any "natural geometry", but in a living connection comparable, or rather identical, with that existing between the parts of my body itself': could we consider the perspective of a child with severe cognitive impairment on this basis?

Sartre (1983: x) stated that 'consciousness is consciousness of something' and distinguished between pre-reflective self-consciousness, where we are aware of ourselves as the recipient of experience, and reflective self-consciousness when we consider our experience as an object in itself. (As an illustration, we could consider the act of being absorbed in reading the previous sentence without being specifically aware of ourself while reading it, and then the pause at the end of the sentence where we consider whether the sentence makes sense and whether we have understood it.) Gallagher discusses the concepts of a 'minimal self', which is a consciousness of oneself as an immediate subject of experience, unextended in time, and the concept of 'non-conceptual first-person content', which is the content of a primitive self-consciousness that is not informed by conceptual thought, such as the content of perception that specifies one's own embodied position in the environment (Gallagher 2011). These concepts involve the idea that 'there is an even more primitive and embodied sense of self than that involved in the use of the first-person pronoun'. A similar approach was advanced by Neisser who described the mutually aware ecological self ('I am the person here in this place, engaged in this particular activity') and the interpersonal self ('I am the person who is engaged, here, in this particular human interchange') (Neisser 1988). Gallagher suggested that these selves were prelinguistic and nonconceptual and were present from birth.

These concepts have been supported by research into neonates who appear from birth, and possibly before birth, to have an organised awareness of their body and their environment, and to be aware of other humans, particularly the mother. In the words of Stern, the world of the 6-week infant is one 'concerned not with how or why something has happened, but with actual, raw experience itself, not with facts or things, but with feelings, his feelings' (Stern 1990). It may be a leap to extrapolate these concepts to the child with severe cerebral palsy, but it would seem that the capacity to experience pleasurable experiences such as warmth, satiety, and human contact, even in a preconceptual and prelinguistic manner, together with the capacity to experience unpleasant experiences such as cold, hunger, isolation, or pain would be in keeping with the presence of a 'minimal self'. This concept does, however, raise a concern; without the development of a narrative self, which allows review and integration of previous experience and allows further development, unpleasant experiences may be even less pleasant as the child may not be able to put them in context or anticipate them.

THE LIVED-IN BODY AS A FOCUS FOR INTERVENTION

Discussion of the child's lived-in or experienced body in the context of their clinical management may initially appear to add another layer of complexity to what is already a complex topic, but does allow a way in which we can consider possible intervention, which is likely to involve the child's objective body, in the context of their lived-in body. From this perspective, an intervention to the child's musculoskeletal system should only be considered if it is likely to improve the child's experience of the world through their lived-in body in comparison to their likely experience without intervention. This may occur in a number of ways:

- through an improvement in a child's capacity to interact more easily with their environment, as may be the case following the provision of powered mobility or by an alteration in the structure of the child's objective body (such as the correction of deformity);
- through the use of assistive devices such as orthoses or walking frames which the child can incorporate into their lived-in body and through which their lived or experienced body may be perceived as needing less control, and in this way being less obtrusive in their experience of the world;
- through the development of improved control of their lived-in body by means of working with each child to make their experienced body less obtrusive;
- through a reduction in any process such as pain which adversely affects their lived experience.

If we see the child's lived-in body as a process, we can appreciate that for each child the adaptive possible, or the potential for improvement or deterioration, will vary and that each child will need to be considered on an individual basis when setting or discussing treatment goals. The concept of the adaptive possible and the potential to cause the child to feel alienated from their own body (as discussed earlier in terms of Sartre's concept of 'my body-for-others') should make us very cautious about the inclusion of normative goals, particularly if these are planned to be achieved through changes in the child's objective body. A view of the child as a process rather than an objective structure, as suggested by Sartre and as suggested by the systems approach discussed earlier, can be positive in that rather than a focus on possible variations from a perceived normative standard in their objective body we can instead see each child as a unique developing system following a particular trajectory while interacting with their world. Our goal as clinicians then becomes to help the child and family to accept this trajectory and to optimise it within the child's adaptive possible while also working with the child and family to optimise the world defined by each child through their lived-in body. In Sartre's terms, this involves helping a child to understand both their facticity, or their given situation, and their capacity for transcendence, namely the degree to which they can surpass this in a way which optimises their experience of the world while avoiding any sense of alienation or embarrassment through comparison with a normative ideal.

This approach may initially appear to reduce the need for clinical evidence and involve a move to a more qualitative approach. This is not the case. The need for clinical evidence to support intervention in this situation is if anything increased, as the goals of intervention will now have a wider focus than those goals which are limited to a change in structure. The approach discussed in the previous chapters regarding an improved understanding of the strengths and limitations of the evidence available for intervention, and the need to critically evaluate what we see as causal pathways in the development and management of musculoskeletal deformity, will remain as essential components of clinical decision-making. The CSH model emphasises the need for all parties to be involved and to make the treatment goals, the evidence for intervention, and the source and validity of this information explicit. The inclusion of a focus on the child's lived-in body and on optimising their experience of their world through their lived-in body may allow this clinical evidence to be more easily apprehended and considered by the child and family.

PUTTING THEORY INTO PRACTICE

The first chapter opened with a discussion of John Cage's composition 4'33". Cage said about this piece that he wanted to remove the focus on the composer and have the listener become aware of their surroundings and to embrace them. In a somewhat similar way, in this book we have moved away from the concept of objective and certain clinical knowledge, which somehow is considered to exist separately from clinicians, to a more interactive and embodied concept of knowledge where the experience of the clinician, like the ambient sounds during a performance of 4'33", influence the clinician's views and where uncertainty is an inevitable consequence of our use of a model to guide and inform management of a complex reality. As discussed above, this does not mean a move towards clinical relativism, where facts or truth depend on the perspective of the observer or on the context in which they occur. We noted in Chapter 1 that Cage said 'my silent piece … expresses the acceptance of whatever happens in that emptiness' (Kostelanetz 2003). In the same way, this approach emphasises the need to both critically appraise the available evidence of a particular clinical approach, as discussed in the previous chapter, and to be aware of the way in which our previous experience and training may influence the way in which we interpret this evidence. All knowledge could be said to depend on the existence of a 'knower'; just as it is not possible to have a piece of music played in a completely silent environment, it is not possible for any of us as clinicians to view evidence from a completely objective perspective free of preconception so to again paraphrase Cage's words our first step as clinicians must be to 'discover a means to let children be themselves rather than vehicles for man-made theories or expressions of human sentiment'. With this is mind, let us look again at the vignettes which were presented at the start of Chapter 1.

Vignette 1: Eleanor

Eleanor is an experienced physiotherapist with a particular interest in the care of children with cerebral palsy. She is attending a clinical case discussion at an international academic meeting regarding possible surgical options for a child with cerebral palsy. Three leading surgeons discuss their preferred options; each surgeon appears confident and seems to view their approach as the most effective one. Eleanor notes that the surgical options advanced by the three surgeons are different. She wonders how each surgeon can be so confident about their approach and why they do not seem concerned that the other surgeons have a different approach. She wonders whether there is an objective 'best approach' or 'best practice', or whether a clinician's approach depends primarily on their experience and training. She wonders also whether the confidence of the surgeons is a response to an awareness of the apparent lack of an agreed and objective approach. She wonders perhaps most of all why the delegates at the meeting seem to accept the discussion and reported that they found it helpful.

Hopefully, having read through the book, the reader will now have a clearer understanding of the factors contributing to this scenario. There are a number of factors which are likely to interact. The opinion advanced by each surgeon will be influenced by their view of the domain in which the clinical scenario is located. If this is considered to be in the 'known' domain, a single therapeutic approach will be considered to represent 'best practice'. If it is in the knowable domain, a number of approaches may be possible within what is considered 'good practice'; the optimal approach can then be considered as possible to identify by means of research such as an RCT. If it is considered to be in the complex domain, the approach may not be clear and will emerge from the interaction between the clinical situation and the surgeon's experience. A potential difficulty may occur when a clinical situation which may be more appropriately placed in the complex domain is instead considered to be in the known or knowable domains; this placement may be influenced by the clinical society in which the knowledge has become externalised. This may lead to a tension between the clinician's implicit clinical knowledge and the explicit knowledge accepted by the society.

In the vignette, each of the three surgeons are making clinical decisions which are valid within each surgeon's own reference frame and which are informed by the boundary judgements that each surgeon has made in this clinical situation. These boundary judgements will be influenced by the experience and the personality of each surgeon. These boundary judgements may be in part a response to an implicitly perceived lack of evidence; in this situation, a clinical opinion may be proffered in a confident manner, which may explain the favourable reception from the audience who are likely themselves to be unsure and keen for a clear approach (or clear approaches!). The expectation within the clinical society of surgeons, particularly those viewed as expert, is likely to include confidence and decisiveness and this may influence how a surgeon will communicate with the clinical society. The acceptance by the audience of the variation between the different surgical recommendations may reflect an implicit acceptance of the complexity of the clinical problem and a perceived validation of an individual flexibility of approach within the explicit guidelines of the clinical society.

Vignette 2: Sue

Sue is a postdoctoral researcher and is an expert on skeletal muscle function. She hopes to become involved in basic science research that will help the care of children with cerebral palsy and has attended a major clinical conference to gain a better understanding of the clinical issues and approach. She appreciates the enthusiasm and commitment of the delegates but is concerned that there appear to be intrinsic contradictions in the accepted treatment model, which essentially involves immobilising and denervating muscle with the aim of helping it to grow. She has noted also that a number of key clinical concepts discussed, such as the concept of spasticity, appear to be incompletely defined when used by the clinicians and appear to have a number of mutually incompatible definitions. She wonders how the clinical model developed and wonders whether the clinicians involved are aware of the inconsistencies within the model. She wonders also whether these issues may limit the development of further understanding of the underlying clinical problem.

From our discussions in this chapter and in previous chapters it would appear that our current clinical model for the management of the musculoskeletal system in children with cerebral palsy is not effective and is more likely to be detrimental than beneficial. Skeletal muscle is generally viewed as a structure, and is assessed by measures such as resistance to stretch and joint passive ranges. Spasticity remains poorly defined, and the concept involves a combination of a clinical sign and a pathophysiological concept. As discussed in Chapter 1, the conflation of these components has resulted in a model where clinicians may consider it possible to treat a perceived pathophysiological entity through intervention to alter a clinical sign. The apparent simplicity of this model, and the apparent attractiveness of the underlying concept, obscure the need to develop our understanding of the complexity of developing biological systems and the associated opportunities for the development of new treatment options aimed at promoting this development.

The degree to which clinicians are aware of inconsistencies within the model is unclear. As discussed in Chapter 1, concern has been expressed about the clinical concept of spasticity, and there are presently a number of conflicting definitions. The concept of spasticity and the associated treatment model have become internalised by clinicians entering the society and have become the 'nomos' which is viewed as objectively true. In a similar manner, the available evidence will be interpreted within a particular clinical paradigm. Thomas Kuhn, who we discussed in Chapter 1, wrote about what he termed 'incommensurability'; by this he meant that a clinician or scientist will work only within a particular paradigm, and will not be able to step outside of this paradigm without accepting an alternative paradigm. Because of this, a clinician or scientist will not be able to compare two paradigms objectively. It may also be helpful to consider the possibility of cognitive dissonance as discussed in Chapter 1; senior clinicians who have invested considerable time and commitment to the development of their practice may not be predisposed to an effective rejection of their treatment approach. This is not suggested as being a conscious process.

Vignette 3: Mobin

Mobin is a physiotherapist looking after Colin, an 8-year-old boy with severe cerebral palsy. Mobin has worked very closely to help Colin to be as comfortable and functional as possible. On the advice of his senior physiotherapy colleagues, he has developed a postural management programme for Colin that involves the use of orthoses, a standing frame, and a sleep system with the aim of correcting Colin's existing lower limb deformities and preventing the development of further deformity. Colin has also had a number of episodes of serial casting and botulinum toxin injections. Mobin and Colin's parents are concerned that Colin appears to be getting stiffer and tighter and that he is finding the use of the orthoses and standing frame uncomfortable. Colin's parents have asked Mobin whether Colin needs to continue with his postural management as it is causing problems with his sleep and his mood. Mobin has previously assumed that this was the best approach but now has concerns that he may not be helping Colin and instead may be making things worse for Colin. He is concerned that if he continues with the present management he may cause Colin more pain, and is concerned that if he stops the present management he may be responsible for allowing Colin's deformities to proceed. He is worried and unsure how to proceed. He notes that his colleagues do not share his concerns and remain convinced of the efficacy of the treatment plan. Mobin wonders if he is missing something.

The present clinical model within the clinical society places Mobin, Colin, and Colin's parents in a difficult position where Colin's treatment-related pain appears to be something that needs to be accepted even though all involved (particularly Colin) are likely to find it distressing. The alternative, which would involve a change in his management programme, may also be perceived as distressing as Mobin and Colin's parents may feel that by inactivity they are contributing to his progression of deformity. Mobin and Colin's parents could use CSH to look at the boundary judgements involved. This would show that the effectiveness of postural management, stretch, and the reduction of muscle activity to optimise musculoskeletal growth is viewed within the clinical society as factual, and that this approach is seen by the clinical society to have value in a clinical situation. The use of this intervention in this situation involves a boundary judgement where the value of intervention aimed at preventing or correcting musculoskeletal deformity is considered as having a higher value than the importance of avoiding discomfort on the part of the child, and where a child's objective body is seen as having more importance or relevance than their lived-in body. A review of the knowledge basis within the CSH framework in regards to the effectiveness of postural management in the correction or prevention of musculo-skeletal deformity would show a lack of evidence to support the use of such an approach. The claim for the effectiveness of this approach, while seen as a fact within the frame of reference of the clinical society, would lack merit for Colin's parents and for Mobin in light of the consequences of the approach in terms of discomfort for Colin without an associated benefit. An alternative approach, involving the use of equipment and orthoses to promote comfort and to facilitate the interaction between Colin's lived-in body and the world in which he is situated, may be seen as having greater merit by Colin's parents and by Mobin (and almost certainly by Colin!) and would represent a way forward for all involved.

Vignette 4: Sara and Miguel

Sara and Miguel are the parents of Maria, a 4-year-old girl with bilateral cerebral palsy. They are concerned about her future independence and mobility. Maria currently takes some steps with the support of a posterior walker, and appears to be making progress in her mobility. Maria's physiotherapist has explained that Maria's walking ability is limited by something called spasticity, which her parents understand causes stiffness and discomfort in Maria's lower limbs and which prevents Maria's muscles from growing as they should. Maria's physiotherapist has discussed a treatment called selective dorsal rhizotomy, which she says can take spasticity away. Maria's parents have been in contact with a team in a hospital in another country who accept international referrals for selective dorsal rhizotomy. This team seem very positive about being able to help Maria to walk independently. Maria's paediatrician has known Maria and her parents since Maria was born and has been very supportive. He has advised caution regarding the potential benefit of selective dorsal rhizotomy for Maria, but when Maria's parents press him for information about Maria's future mobility, he does not seem to be able to give them the precise and definite prediction that they feel they need to be able to plan ahead. The treatment is very expensive, and it means putting Maria through surgery and extensive rehabilitation afterwards, but it seems to offer Maria the ability to walk independently. Maria's parents trust her paediatrician but he seems to be less positive in his approach than the team in the hospital and less definite about the outcome of surgery for Maria. The explanation from Maria's physiotherapist about the role and importance of spasticity makes sense to her parents and the positive approach of the surgical team is encouraging. Surely the team in the specialist hospital would not be as positive unless the treatment really worked as they said?

Sara, Miguel, and the clinicians involved in this vignette will all have Maria's best interests at heart but will all have a particular bias or perspective. The positive and apparently clear message of the physiotherapist and the team in the international centre will be more likely to be accepted by the parents than the less clear and less positive approach of the paediatrician, but is likely to be influenced both by a strong desire to help on the part of the clinicians and, potentially for the team in the referral centre, by a degree of cognitive dissonance. The approach focuses on intervention to an impairment with the aim of bringing Maria closer to typical development; Maria's objective body is the focus rather than her lived-in body. This scenario would be very suitable for CSH, but this approach may not be acceptable to everyone involved: for the parents it may mean a less positive message and treatment outcome, and for the physiotherapist and the team in the hospital it will involve a critical appraisal of their treatment model.

Vignette 5: Ana

Ana is a children's orthopaedic surgeon who has been monitoring the hip development of Peter, a 5-year-old boy with bilateral cerebral palsy. Peter has mild hip dysplasia, which does not appear to be progressing, and has significant medical comorbidities including problems with epilepsy, respiratory function, and gastro-oesophageal reflux. Ana's view has been that the risks of surgical intervention to his hips for Peter at present outweigh the likely benefits, and she has explained this to Peter's parents, Tom and Mary. They have been asking Ana for definite predictions about Peter's hips both in terms of his likelihood of progression of dysplasia and his risk of long-term hip pain. Ana has explained that this is difficult to precisely quantify. Tom and Mary have now contacted Ana to say that Tom will be having bilateral hip surgery done by another surgeon in a different hospital, following their request for a second surgical opinion. Tom and Mary have explained that the other surgeon seemed more confident and much more definite about what was likely to happen to Peter's hips without surgery, and showed them clear guidelines about the management of hip dysplasia in children with cerebral palsy. Ana is an experienced surgeon who has kept up to date with the published literature on hip dysplasia in children with cerebral palsy. She wonders why things do not seem as clear for her as they seemed to the other surgeon and wonders why she finds it difficult to give definite predictions of the natural history of hip dysplasia and the outcome of surgery for an individual child.

This vignette shares some of the features seen in the previous vignettes and has been covered also in the section on CSH in this chapter. It is likely that Ana views hip dysplasia as being located in the complex domain, where accurate prediction in an individual is difficult and where practice is emergent. The other surgeon may view hip dysplasia as being located in the known domain where there is best practice and where the guidelines are clear. Like surgeons, parents are not all alike and some parents may be more accepting of uncertainty than others. A relevant factor here may be the type of uncertainty in question, whether epistemic, aleatory, or ontologic. Epistemic uncertainty occurs when we do not have all of the information which is available; this uncertainty can be reduced in a clinical situation. Aleatory uncertainty relates to outcomes which cannot be predicted such as the throw of a dice. This type of uncertainty will be inevitable to an extent when making predictions about a biological system and will be assumed as inherent if the clinical situation is thought to be in the complex domain. Ontologic uncertainty refers to aspects of a situation which are not known, namely those aspects which we do not know what we do not know. Ontologic and aleatory uncertainty, however, will be viewed as unnecessary if the clinical situation is thought to be in the known or knowable domains. It is possible for clinicians that uncertainty is initially viewed predominantly as epistemic, and that with increasing clinical experience and with an associated reduction in epistemic uncertainty there is an increasing awareness of aleatory and ontologic uncertainty.

Vignette 6: Hans

Hans is a 12-year-old boy with bilateral cerebral palsy. He finds it increasingly difficult to walk with the support of his posterior walker; his legs become tired and uncomfortable, and his splints feel heavy. Hans has just started at secondary school and finds this difficult. The school is larger than his previous school and he has not made many friends yet. Hans feels self-conscious when he walks and thinks that people are looking at him. He finds his wheelchair is comfortable and finds it easier to get around in his wheelchair, but his parents and physiotherapist are keen for him to walk as much as he can.

Hans feels that he has had a lot done to his legs including physiotherapy, splinting, casting, botulinum toxin injections, and surgery. He has daily stretches, which are uncomfortable. His physiotherapist and his parents talk to him about 'spasticity' and 'core strength', and are discussing the use of a standing frame to stretch his legs and about the possibility of more surgery. Hans' friend Stella had surgery recently because she did not like the way her legs looked and because she thought that she might make friends more easily if her legs looked better and worked better. Stella has told Hans that her legs look straighter now, but she still has problems walking and still finds it hard to make friends. Hans does not think that he wants any more surgery. Hans knows that his parents and physiotherapist want to help him but wonders why everyone seems more interested in his legs than in him.

The degree to which a child will become involved in clinical decision-making will be influenced by the child's age and cognitive level, but as discussed earlier in this chapter, the child will always have their own perspective, and consideration of clinical management without incorporation of the perspective of the child may not be helpful. As clinicians, we are by definition limited to direct assessment of the child's objective body; an understanding of the child's lived-in body and hence an understanding of the problems faced by the child and the potential impact of intervention can be achieved only through discussion and interaction with the child. If a focus on assessment and management of the child's objective body means that their lived-in body becomes less important to us, to their family, or to the child, then our clinical practice is not optimal. In Merleau-Ponty's words (2002: 177) 'our body is not the object of an "I think": it is an ensemble of lived meanings that finds its equilibrium'. Our role as clinicians is to identify how we can help the child improve these lived meanings. This may be possible through intervention or may be possible through helping the child and family to move away from normative goals.

DOES LIFE REALLY NEED TO BE THIS COMPLICATED?

At first viewing, the approach outlined in this chapter may seem unduly complex and may seem to lack the apparent directness and simplicity of our current clinical model. Mixing systems theory and existentialism can seem unnecessarily confusing but can be considered as looking at the same central complex phenomenon, namely the lived experience of a child with cerebral palsy, from different perspectives. Such an approach recognises and accepts our limited understanding of musculoskeletal growth and development in children with cerebral palsy, and our awareness of the variability involved, while also recognising that there is a level of shared understanding and there is evidence available to guide our clinical management. This approach does not reduce the necessity for evidence, and instead emphasises the need for critical appraisal of evidence and an awareness of potential sources of error or of bias. It allows us to place this appraised evidence within the context of a broader clinical model which views the musculoskeletal system within an overall system of nested interacting systems ranging from the cell to the child and from the child to the community. The impact of intervention to alter structure or to alter what is seen as an impairment may not be predictable; the goal of intervention may instead be best considered through its potential to improve the child's experience of their world through their lived-in body. This involves a shift in clinical perspective, as to optimise how a child experiences the world in this way will need greater understanding of how the child experiences their world. In the words of Mulderij (2000):

> We are not only treating a moving body, we are treating a child who is out to explore the world physically, to enjoy freedom of action, and to confer his or her own meanings on the world.

Perhaps most importantly, this approach allows us to see each child's lived-in body not as objectively closer to or farther away from an abstract normative ideal but instead as a combination of a unique complex adaptive system and a unique lived-in body through which the world and other people in the world are experienced by the child. Our challenges as clinicians are to understand more about the experienced world of the child, to understand how the child's objective body contributes to this experience, to understand the individual adaptive potential of each child, and to both critically appraise existing evidence and develop new evidence to support interventions which are life and world-enhancing for the child.

This is not a new concept or approach. We saw earlier in this chapter during the discussion about Hippocrates' first aphorism that the term paediatrics comes from the Greek words 'pais', a child, and 'iatros', a healer. Iatros in turn comes from the Greek verb 'iomai', to heal or make whole. Paediatrics can thus be translated as 'making children whole'. The concept of healing or making whole predates Hippocrates; the Greek term iatros, used by Hippocrates over 2000 years ago, is thought to have been derived from earlier languages including Babylonian and has been traced back 2000 years earlier to the word 'a-zu' or 'healer' in the earliest written language, Sumerian (Martin 2009). The root 'zu' in Sumerian comes from a verb meaning to know, experience, or understand . When we say 'paediatrics', we are using a word meaning an association between experience, knowledge, and healing or making children whole that has existed at least since the earliest written language more than 4000 years ago. For the child with cerebral palsy, the concepts of 'healing' or 'making whole' transcend any arbitrary normative connotation and paradoxically move instead towards a focus on supporting each child to see themselves as they are: already whole, and not in need of healing.

Conclusion
Putting it Into Practice

There is a (possibly apocryphal) story of a tourist asking for directions to a nearby town. 'Well', came the response, 'If I were you I wouldn't start from here at all.' Having reached the end of the book, you may also wonder if this is the best place to start. In place of a widely accepted and apparently clear clinical model with clear clinical goals, we have advocated embracing complexity, uncertainty, and an awareness that any clinical model involves a simplification of this complexity. You will hopefully be aware of the potential benefits of this approach, which include improved understanding and a move away from a normative approach to treatment outcomes, but may be less clear about how to implement such an approach in your clinical practise or research.

The first step is to accept that, in the words of the physicist Werner Heisenberg, 'the universe is not only stranger than we think but stranger than we can think'. As discussed in Chapter 6, clinical models are at best a simplification or approximation of the underlying complex reality but despite this are essential in dealing with this complex reality. The key is to develop a useful and effective model while remaining aware of the limitations of the model. This can be helped by ensuring that the concepts used in the model are clear and are defined in a manner that is consistent with their usage in the model. As discussed in Chapter 1, it may be helpful also to distinguish between the 'percept', the data which we obtain through experience or assessment, and the 'concept', which refers to how we interpret the information. As an example, the percept of a resistance to passive stretch of a muscle on clinical examination is more informative and less confusing than the concept of spasticity.

It may also be helpful to be explicit about how you consider causation in your model through the use of causal loop diagrams in Chapter 4 and causal structure diagrams as discussed in Chapter 5. These diagrams do not need to be complex; the level of complexity involved will depend on the complexity of the model. Causal diagrams can, however, suggest how the hypotheses used to inform the model may be tested experimentally. These causal structures and hypotheses could be included in the introduction section of any publication so that the reader can appreciate the underlying model used. As discussed in Chapter 1, such a model will guide research until it is superseded by a newer model which may not be more 'correct' but may be more effective in helping us work with the available data.

Inclusion of the causal structures on which a model is based may be particularly helpful in the design and interpretation of RCTs as discussed in Chapter 4; this in turn may allow inclusion of biological outcomes to test the effectiveness of the clinical model. Inclusion of causal structures, hypotheses, and biological outcomes may be particularly important in grant applications where they could be combined with the inclusion on the grant awards panel of scientists with the relevant biological expertise.

In this book, we have suggested that, in many cases, empirical evidence may be insufficient on its own to support an intervention, particularly when there is heterogeneity in the response of participants. Clinical guidance committees should include basic scientists to describe mechanisms by which the intervention may be successful, and to help identify in which participants the intervention may be most effective. In this way, guidance in the context of uncertainty may be more nuanced and more useful to the clinical practitioner, allowing them to exercise their understanding of the individual patient in their clinic.

Considering the child's musculoskeletal system as a complex system with a particular trajectory within a state space, as discussed in Chapter 6, opens the possibility of defining and hence predicting the range of possible trajectories of development of a system. This moves us away from normative goals towards the musculoskeletal system's 'adaptive possible', namely the capacity for alteration in development or trajectory in the system. Modelling of such a system is complex, but recent developments in causal inference in nonlinear systems mean this is a realisable goal (e.g. Runge et al. 2019). An improved understanding of system development in an individual would reduce the difficulties discussed in Chapter 5 in predicting individual outcome on the basis of available evidence.

Along with hypotheses and potential causal mechanisms, the goals of intervention should be made explicit in any clinical model as should whom and what we are treating. To use Sartre's concepts as discussed in Chapter 6, we need to clarify whether our treatment is aimed at benefiting the child's experienced body, their objective body, or their body-for-others. It may be that bringing about an improvement in the child's experience of the world through an alteration in their experienced or lived-in body may need to be brought about through an alteration in their objective body, but the links and potential causative mechanisms implied in this model need to be clarified and made explicit before we consider intervention. It is in this area where the concepts we discussed regarding clinical knowledge, evidence, causation, and complex adaptive systems become most relevant to the clinician, child, and family, and where the possibility of new models and new therapeutic approaches offer exciting future opportunities to improve the child's interaction with, and experience of, the world of which they are a part.

References

Aarts PB, Jongerius PH, Geerdink YA, van Limbeek J, Geurts AC (2010) Effectiveness of modified constraint-induced movement therapy in children with unilateral spastic cerebral palsy: a randomized controlled trial. *Neurorehabilitation and Neural Repair* **24**(6): 509–518. doi: 10.1177/1545968309359767.

Abadi A, Glover EI, Isfort RJ et al. (2009) Limb immobilization induces a coordinate down-regulation of mitochondrial and other metabolic pathways in men and women. *PloS One* **4**(8): e6518.

Adami C (2016) What is information? *Philosophical Transactions of the Royal Society A: Mathematical, Physical and Engineering Sciences* **374**(2063): 20150230.

Agbulut O, Noirez P, Beaumont F et al. (2003) Myosin heavy chain isoforms in postnatal muscle development of mice. *Biology of the Cell* **95**(6): 399–406. doi: 10.1016/s0248-4900(03)00087-x.

Anglemyer A, Horvath HT, Bero L (2014) Healthcare outcomes assessed with observational study designs compared with those assessed in randomized trials. *Cochrane Database of Systematic Reviews* **2014**(4): MR000034. doi: 10.1002/14651858.MR000034.pub2.

Arber S, Costa RM (2018) Connecting neuronal circuits for movement. *Science* **360**(6396): 1403–1404.

Aristotle (2004) *The Nicomachean Ethics.* London: Penguin Books.

Arnould C, Penta M, Renders A, Thonnard JL (2004) ABILHAND-Kids: a measure of manual ability in children with cerebral palsy. *Neurology* **63**(6): 1045–1052. doi: 10.1212/01.wnl.0000138423.77640.37.

Atherton PJ, Szewczyk NJ, Selby A et al. (2009) Cyclic stretch reduces myofibrillar protein synthesis despite increases in FAK and anabolic signalling in L6 cells. *The Journal of Physiology* **587**(Pt 14): 3719–3727. doi: 10.1113/jphysiol.2009.169854.

Azeloglu EU, Iyengar R (2015) Signaling networks: information flow, computation, and decision making. *Cold Spring Harbor Perspectives in Biology* **7**(4): a005934.

Baker JS, McCormick MC, Robergs RA (2010) Interaction among skeletal muscle metabolic energy systems during intense exercise. *Journal of Nutrition and Metabolism* **2010**: 905612. doi: 10.1155/2010/905612.

Barber L, Hastings-Ison T, Baker R, Barrett R, Lichtwark G (2011) Medial gastrocnemius muscle volume and fascicle length in children aged 2 to 5 years with cerebral palsy. *Developmental Medicine and Child Neurology* **53**(6): 543–548. doi: 10.1111/j.1469-8749.2011.03913.x.

Baron RM, Kenny DA (1986) The moderator-mediator variable distinction in social psychological research: conceptual, strategic, and statistical considerations. *Journal of Personality and Social Psychology* **51**(6): 1173–1182. doi: 10.1037//0022-3514.51.6.1173.

Barraclough K (2004) Why doctors don't read research papers. *British Medical Journal* **329**: 1411.

Bedi KS, Birzgalis AR, Mahon M, Smart JL, Wareham AC (1982) Early life undernutrition in rats. 1. Quantitative histology of skeletal muscles from underfed young and refed adult animals. *The British Journal of Nutrition* **47**(3): 417–431. doi: 10.1079/bjn19820053.

Benard MR, Harlaar J, Becher JG, Huijing PA, Jaspers RT (2011) Effects of growth on geometry of gastrocnemius muscle in children: a three-dimensional ultrasound analysis. *Journal of Anatomy* **219**(3): 388–402. doi: 10.1111/j.1469-7580.2011.01402.x.

Berger PL (1967) *The Sacred Canopy: Elements of a Sociological Theory of Religion.* New York: Doubleday and Company.

Berger PL, Luckmann T (1991) *The Social Construction of Reality: A Treatise in the Sociology of Knowledge*. London: Penguin.

Biering-Sorensen B, Kristensen IB, Kjaer M, Biering-Sorensen F (2009) Muscle after spinal cord injury. *Muscle & Nerve* **40**(4): 499–519. doi: 10.1002/mus.21391.

Binkley T, Johnson J, Vogel L, Kecskemethy H, Henderson R, Specker B (2005) Bone measurements by peripheral quantitative computed tomography (pQCT) in children with cerebral palsy. *The Journal of Pediatrics* **147**(6): 791–796. doi: 10.1016/j.jpeds.2005.07.014.

Bjornson K, Hays R, Graubert C et al. (2007) Botulinum toxin for spasticity in children with cerebral palsy: a comprehensive evaluation. *Pediatrics* **120**(1): 49–58. doi: 10.1542/peds.2007-0016.

BMJ (1948) Streptomycin in Tuberculosis Trials Committee. *Br Med J* **2**: 769. doi: 10.1136/bmj.2.4582.769.

Boël G, Danot O, de Lorenzo V et al. (2019) Omnipresent Maxwell's demons orchestrate information management in living cells. *Microbial Biotechnology* **12**(2): 210–242.

Box GEP (1979) Robustness in the strategy of scientific model building. In: Launer RL, Wilkinson GN, editors, *Robustness in Statistics*. Cambridge, MA: Academic Press, pp. 201–236.

Boyd RN, Graham HK (1999) Objective measurement of clinical findings in the use of botulinum toxin type A for the management of children with cerebral palsy. *European Journal of Neurology* **6**(suppl 4): s23–s35. doi: 10.1111/j.1468-1331.1999.tb00031.x.

Brameld JM, Buttery PJ, Dawson JM, Harper JMM (1998) Nutritional and hormonal control of skeletal-muscle cell growth and differentiation. *The Proceedings of the Nutrition Society* **57**(2): 207–217. doi: 10.1079/pns19980033.

Brenner S (1999) Theoretical biology in the third millennium. *Philosophical Transactions of the Royal Society* **354**(1392): 1963–1965.

Brown CS, Bachmann GA, Foster DC (2013) Challenge of conducting a multicenter clinical trial: experience in commencing a vulvodynia research protocol. *Journal of Women's Health* **2002**: 291–292. doi: 10.1089/jwh.2013.4281.

Cage J (1961) *Silence: Lectures and Writings*. Hanover: Wesleyan University Press.

Cage J (1968) Interview by John Kobler, 'Everything We Do Is Music', *Saturday Evening Post*, quoted in Richard Kostelanetz (1988) *Conversing with Cage*. New York: Limelight Editions, p. 65.

Cage J (1990) *Autobiographical Statement*. [online] Available at: https://johncage.org/autobiographical_statement.html [Accessed 26 July 2021].

Carroll L (1871) Through the looking-glass, and what Alice found there. Accessed through Project Gutenberg on 31 October 2021 at https://www.gutenberg.org/cache/epub/12/pg12-images.html#link2HCH0006.

Chakrabarty S, Martin JH (2000) Postnatal development of the motor representation in primary motor cortex. *Journal of Neurophysiology* **84**(5): 2582–2594. doi: 10.1152/jn.2000.84.5.2582.

Chakrabarty S, Martin JH (2010) Postnatal development of a segmental switch enables corticospinal tract transmission to spinal forelimb motor circuits. *The Journal of Neuroscience* **30**(6): 2277–2288. doi: 10.1523/JNEUROSCI.5286-09.2010.

Christlieb IY, Cesarman E (1996) Thermodynamics of skeletal muscle fiber: do we need to redefine 'active' and 'resting' states. *BAM-PADOVA* **6**: 199–202.

Chugh R (2015) Do Australian universities encourage tacit knowledge transfer? *KMIS* **3**: 128–135.

Clarke RD (1946) An application of the Poisson distribution. *Journal of the Institute of Actuaries* **72**(3): 481.

Clemmons DR (2009) Role of IGF-I in skeletal muscle mass maintenance. *Trends in Endocrinology and Metabolism* **20**(7): 349–356. doi: 10.1016/j.tem.2009.04.002.

Clowry GJ (2007) The dependence of spinal cord development on corticospinal input and its significance in understanding and treating spastic cerebral palsy. *Neuroscience and Biobehavioral Reviews* **31**(8): 1114–1124. doi: 10.1016/j.neubiorev.2007.04.007.

Clowry GJ, Walker L, Davies P (2006) The effects of botulinum neurotoxin A induced muscle paresis during a critical period upon muscle and spinal cord development in the rat. *Experimental Neurology* **202**(2): 456–469. doi: 10.1016/j.expneurol.2006.07.008.

Cohen J (1992) A power primer. *Psychological Bulletin* **112**(1): 155–159. doi: 10.1037//0033-2909.112.1.155.

Cole J, Inahara M, Peckitt M (2017) First person accounts of cerebral palsy: adding phenomenological to medical and social models of chronic conditions. *SM Journal of Neurology and Neuroscience* **3**(3): 1016s1.

Coleman-Fountain E, McLaughlin J (2013) The interactions of disability and impairment. *Social Theory & Health* **11**(2): 133–150.

Cook CE (2008) Clinimetrics corner: the Minimal Clinically Important Change Score (MCID): a necessary pretense. *Journal of Manual & Manipulative Therapy* **16**(4): 82E–83E. doi: 10.1179/jmt.2008.16.4.82e.

Cooke PH, Cole WG, Carey RP (1989) Dislocation of the hip in cerebral palsy. Natural history and predictability. *The Journal of Bone and Joint Surgery* **71**(3): 441–446. doi: 10.1302/0301-620X.71B3.2722938.

Coq JO, Xerri C (1999) Tactile impoverishment and sensorimotor restriction deteriorate the forepaw cutaneous map in the primary somatosensory cortex of adult rats. *Experimental Brain Research* **129**(4): 518–531. doi: 10.1007/s002210050922.

Corr A, Smith J, Baldock P (2017) Neuronal control of bone remodeling. *Toxicologic Pathology* **45**(7): 894–903.

Crabtree NJ, Kibirige MS, Fordham JN et al. (2004) The relationship between lean body mass and bone mineral content in paediatric health and disease. *Bone* **35**(4): 965–972. doi: 10.1016/j.bone.2004.06.009.

Croskerry P (2002) Achieving quality in clinical decision making: cognitive strategies and detection of bias. *Academic Emergency Medicine* **9**(11): 1184–1204. doi: 10.1111/j.1553-2712.2002.tb01574.x.

Cummings E (1991) *Complete Poems (1904–1962)*. Edited by Firmage G. New York: Liveright Publishing Corporation.

Davies JA (2014) *Life Unfolding: How the Human Body Creates Itself.* Oxford: Oxford University Press.

Davies PSW, Ewing G, Lucas A (1989) Energy expenditure in early infancy. *British Journal of Nutrition* **62**(3): 621–629.

Davies P (2020) *The Demon in the Machine: How Hidden Webs of Information Are Finally Solving the Mystery of Life.* London: Penguin Books.

Dayanidhi S, Buckner EH, Redmond RS, Chambers HG, Schenk S, Lieber RL (2021) Skeletal muscle maximal mitochondrial activity in ambulatory children with cerebral palsy. *Developmental Medicine and Child Neurology* **63**(10): 1194–1203. doi: 10.1111/dmcn.14785.

Deacon T, Koutroufinis S (2014) Complexity and dynamical depth. *Information* **5**(3): 404–423.

Deci EL, Ryan RM (2000) The 'what' and 'why' of goal pursuits: human needs and the self-determination of behavior. *Psychological Inquiry* **11**(4): 227–268. doi: 10.1207/S15327965PLI1104_01.

Dennett DC (2013) *Intuition Pumps and Other Tools for Thinking.* New York: WW Norton & Company.

Derrida J (1977) Limited Inc. Evanston, IL: Northwestern University Press, 136.

Domenighetti AA, Mathewson MA, Pichika R et al. (2018) Loss of myogenic potential and fusion capacity of muscle stem cells isolated from contracted muscle in children with cerebral palsy. *American Journal of Physiology. Cell Physiology* **315**(2): C247–C257. doi: 10.1152/ajpcell.00351.2017.

Dort J, Fabre P, Molina T, Dumont N (2019) Macrophages are key regulators of stem cells during skeletal muscle regeneration and diseases. *Stem Cells International* **2019**. https://doi.org/10.1155/2019/4761427.

Duckworth W (1989) Anything I say will be misunderstood: an interview with John Cage. In: Fleming R, Duckworth W, editors, *John Cage at Seventy-Five.* Cranbury, NJ; London; and Ontario, Canada: Associated University Presses, pp. 21–22.

Eames NW, Baker R, Hill N, Graham K, Taylor T, Cosgrove A (1999) The effect of botulinum toxin A on gastrocnemius length: magnitude and duration of response. *Developmental Medicine and Child Neurology* **41**(4): 226–232. doi: 10.1017/S0012162299000493.

Eken T, Elder GCB, Lømo T (2008) Development of tonic firing behavior in rat soleus muscle. *Journal of Neurophysiology* **99**(4): 1899–1905. doi: 10.1152/jn.00834.2007.

Elstein AS, Schwartz A (2002) Clinical problem solving and diagnostic decision making: selective review of the cognitive literature. *BMJ (Clinical Research Ed.)* **324**(7339): 729–732. doi: 10.1136/bmj.324.7339.729.

Feher J (2017) *Quantitative Human Physiology: An Introduction.* Cambridge, MA: Academic Press. https://doi.org/10.1016/B978-0-12-800883-6.00095-1.

Fenollosa E (1920) *Instigations of Ezra Pound together with an Essay on the Chinese Written Character by Ernest Fenollosa.* New York: Boni and Liveright. https://www.gutenberg.org/files/40852/40852-h/40852-h.htm.

Festinger L, Riecken H, Schachter S (2017) *When Prophecy Fails: A Social and Psychological Study of a Modern Group That Predicted the Destruction of the World.* Morrisville, NC: Lulu Press, Inc.

Fleck L (1979) *Genesis and Development of a Scientific Fact.* Chicago: University of Chicago Press.

Forssberg H (1985) Ontogeny of human locomotor control. I. Infant stepping, supported locomotion and transition to independent locomotion. *Experimental Brain Research* **57**(3): 480–493. doi: 10.1007/BF00237835.

Fosang AL, Galea MP, McCoy AT, Reddihough DS, Story I (2003) Measures of muscle and joint performance in the lower limb of children with cerebral palsy. *Developmental Medicine and Child Neurology* **45**(10): 664–670. doi: 10.1017/s0012162203001245.

Fulco M, Cen Y, Zhao P et al. (2008) Glucose restriction inhibits skeletal myoblast differentiation by activating SIRT1 through AMPK-mediated regulation of Nampt. *Developmental Cell* **14**(5): 661–673. doi: 10.1016/j.devcel.2008.02.004.

Gallagher S, editor, (2011) *The Oxford Handbook of the Self.* Oxford: Oxford University.

Gao T, Díaz-Hirashi Z, Verdeguer F (2018) Metabolic signaling into chromatin modifications in the regulation of gene expression. *International Journal of Molecular Sciences* **19**(12). doi: 10.3390/ijms19124108.

Gibson CL, Clowry GJ (1999) Retraction of muscle afferents from the rat ventral horn during development. *Neuroreport* **10**(2): 231–235. doi: 10.1097/00001756-199902050-00006.

Glancy B, Hartnell LM, Malide D et al. (2015) Mitochondrial reticulum for cellular energy distribution in muscle. *Nature* **523**(7562): 617–620. doi: 10.1038/nature14614.

Glover EI, Phillips SM, Oates BR et al. (2008) Immobilization induces anabolic resistance in human myofibrillar protein synthesis with low and high dose amino acid infusion. *The Journal of Physiology* **586**(24): 6049–6061.

Gomes AR, Soares AG, Peviani S, Nascimento RB, Moriscot AS, Salvini TF (2006) The effect of 30 minutes of passive stretch of the rat soleus muscle on the myogenic differentiation, myostatin, and atrogin-1 gene expressions. *Archives of Physical Medicine and Rehabilitation* **87**(2): 241–246. doi: 10.1016/j.apmr.2005.08.126.

Gramsbergen A, Ijkema-Paasen J, Nikkels PGJ, Hadders-Algra M (1997) Regression of polyneural innervation in the human psoas muscle. *Early Human Development* **49**(1): 49–61. doi: 10.1016/s0378-3782(97)01876-8.

Greene JA, Podolsky SH (2012) Reform, regulation, and pharmaceuticals – the Kefauver-Harris Amendments at 50. *The New England Journal of Medicine* **367**(16): 1481–1483. doi: 10.1056/NEJMp1210007.

Gundersen K (2011) Excitation-transcription coupling in skeletal muscle: the molecular pathways of exercise. *Biological Reviews of the Cambridge Philosophical Society* **86**(3): 564–600. doi: 10.1111/j.1469-185X.2010.00161.x.

Harold FM (2001) *The Way of the Cell: Molecules, Organisms, and the Order of Life*. Oxford: Oxford University Press.

Harris JJ, Attwell D (2012) The energetics of CNS white matter. *The Journal of Neuroscience* **32**(1): 356–371. doi: 10.1523/JNEUROSCI.3430-11.2012.

Harvey A, Caretti G, Moresi V, Renzini A, Adamo S (2019) Interplay between metabolites and the epigenome in regulating embryonic and adult stem cell potency and maintenance. *Stem Cell Reports* **13**: 573–598.

Hay WW, Thureen P (2010) Protein for preterm infants: how much is needed? How much is enough? How much is too much? *Pediatrics and Neonatology* **51**(4): 198–207. doi: 10.1016/S1875-9572(10)60039-3.

Hayashi T, Stuchebrukhov AA (2011) Quantum electron tunneling in respiratory complex I. *The Journal of Physical Chemistry B* **115**(18): 5354–5364. doi: 10.1021/jp109410j.

Head ML, Holman L, Lanfear R, Kahn AT, Jennions MD (2015) The extent and consequences of p-hacking in science. *PLoS Biology* **13**(3): 1–15. doi: 10.1371/journal.pbio.1002106.

Heinonen A, McKay HA, Whittall KP, Forster BB, Khan KM (2001) Muscle cross-sectional area is associated with specific site of bone in prepubertal girls: a quantitative magnetic resonance imaging study. *Bone* **29**(4): 388–392. doi: 10.1016/s8756-3282(01)00588-9.

Henneman E, Olson CB (1965) Relations between structure and function in the design of skeletal muscles. *Journal of Neurophysiology* **28**: 581–598. doi: 10.1152/jn.1965.28.3.581.

Hermanson M, Hagglund G, Riad J, Rodby-Bousquet E, Wagner P (2015) Prediction of hip displacement in children with cerebral palsy: development of the CPUP hip score. *The Bone & Joint Journal* **97**(10): 1441–1444.

Herskind A, Ritterband-Rosenbaum A, Willerslev-Olsen M et al. (2016) Muscle growth is reduced in 15-month-old children with cerebral palsy. *Developmental Medicine and Child Neurology* **58**(5): 485–491. doi: 10.1111/dmcn.12950.

Hill AB (2005) The environment and disease: association or causation? *Bulletin of the World Health Organization* **83**(10): 295–300.

Hoffmann C, Weigert C (2017) Skeletal muscle as an endocrine organ: the role of myokines in exercise adaptations. *Cold Spring Harbor Perspectives in Medicine* **7**(11): a029793. doi: 10.1101/cshperspect.a029793.

Hoon AH, Stashinko EE, Nagae LM et al. (2009) Sensory and motor deficits in children with cerebral palsy born preterm correlate with diffusion tensor imaging abnormalities in thalamocortical pathways. *Developmental Medicine and Child Neurology* **51**(9): 697–704. doi: 10.1111/j.1469-8749.2009.03306.x.

Huang S (2010) Cell lineage determination in state space: a systems view brings flexibility to dogmatic canonical rules. *PLoS Biology* **8**(5): e1000380. doi: 10.1371/journal.pbio.1000380.

Huang S, Wikswo J (2006) Dimensions of systems biology. *Reviews of Physiology Biochemistry and Pharmacology* **2006**: 81–104.

Hughes MA, Myers BS, Schenkman ML (1996) The role of strength in rising from a chair in the functionally impaired elderly. *Journal of Biomechanics* **29**(12): 1509–1513. doi: 10.1016/S0021-9290(96)80001-7.

Husserl E (1970) *Logical Investigations*. New York: Routledge & Kegan Paul.

Ijkema-Paassen J, Gramsbergen A (2005) Development of postural muscles and their innervation. *Neural Plasticity* **12**(2–3): 141–151. doi: 10.1155/NP.2005.141.

Irvine B, Green DG. (2002) Social insurance the right way forward for health care in the United Kingdom? *British Medical Journal* **325**(7362): 488. doi: 10.1136/bmj.325.7362.488.

Isaacs D, Fitzgerald D (1999) Seven alternatives to evidence based medicine. *BMJ (Clinical Research Ed.)* **319**(7225): 1618. doi: 10.1136/bmj.319.7225.1618.

Jooyeon K, MinYoung K (2013) Reliability and responsiveness of the Gross Motor Function Measure-88 in children with cerebral palsy. *Physical Therapy* **93**(3): 393–400. doi: https://doi.org/10.2522/ptj.20110374.

Kacser H, Waddington CH (1957) *The Strategy of the Genes.* London: Allen and Unwin.

Kahneman D (2011) *Thinking, Fast and Slow.* London: Macmillan.

Kajimura D, Lee HW, Riley KJ et al. (2013) Adiponectin regulates bone mass via opposite central and peripheral mechanisms through FoxO1. *Cell Metabolism* **17**(6): 901–915. doi: 10.1016/j.cmet.2013.04.009.

Karsenty G, Olson EN (2016) Bone and muscle endocrine functions: unexpected paradigms of inter-organ communication. *Cell* **164**(6): 1248–1256. doi: 10.1016/j.cell.2016.02.043.

Kauffman SA (1993) *The Origins of Order: Self-organization and Selection in Evolution.* New York: Oxford University Press.

Kerr NL (1998) HARKing: hypothesizing after the results are known. *Personality and Social Psychology Review* **2**(3): 196–217.

Klingels K, Jaspers E, Van de Winckel A, De Cock P, Molenaers G, Feys H (2010) A systematic review of arm activity measures for children with hemiplegic cerebral palsy. *Clinical Rehabilitation* **24**(10): pp. 887–900.

Kim H, Davies P, Walker SI (2015) New scaling relation for information transfer in biological networks. *Journal of the Royal Society Interface* **12**(113): 20150944.

Kim HM, Galatz LM, Das R, Patel N, Thomopoulos S (2009) Recovery potential after postnatal shoulder paralysis. An animal model of neonatal brachial plexus palsy. *The Journal of Bone and Joint Surgery* **91**(4): 879–891. doi: 10.2106/JBJS.H.00088.

Kokol P, Završnik J, Vošner HB (2017) Artificial intelligence and pediatrics: a synthetic mini review. *Pediatr Dimensions* **2**(4): 1–5. doi: 10.15761/PD.1000155.

Kollias HD, McDermott JC (2008) Transforming growth factor-beta and myostatin signaling in skeletal muscle. *Journal of Applied Physiology* **104**(3): 579–587. doi: 10.1152/japplphysiol.01091.2007.

Kostelanetz R (2003) *Conversing with Cage,* 2nd edn. New York: Taylor and Francis. Available at: https://www.perlego.com/book/1614239/conversing-with-cage-pdf [Accessed: 31 October 2021].

Kraemer HC, Kupfer DJ (2006) Size of treatment effects and their importance to clinical research and practice. *Biological Psychiatry* **59**(11): 990–996. doi: 10.1016/j.biopsych.2005.09.014.

Krumlinde-Sundholm L, Holmefur M, Kottorp A, Eliasson AC (2007) The Assisting Hand Assessment: current evidence of validity, reliability, and responsiveness to change. *Developmental Medicine and Child Neurology* **49**(4): 259–264. doi: 10.1111/j.1469-8749.2007.00259.x.

Kuhn T (1970) *The Structure of Scientific Revolutions,* 2nd edn. Chicago: University of Chicago Press.

Kurtz CF, Snowden DJ (2003) The new dynamics of strategy: sense-making in a complex and complicated world. *IBM Systems Journal* **42**(3): 462–483.

Kuzawa CW, Chugani HT, Grossman LI et al. (2014) Metabolic costs and evolutionary implications of human brain development. *Proceedings of the National Academy of Sciences of the United States of America* **111**(36): 13010–13015. doi: 10.1073/pnas.1323099111.

Lance JW (1980) The control of muscle tone, reflexes and movement: the Robert Wartenberg lecture. *Neurology* **30**(12): 1303. doi: 10.1212/WNL.30.12.1303.

Lance JW (1990) What is spasticity? *Lancet* **335**(8689): 606. doi: 10.1016/0140-6736(90)90389-m.

Laplante M, Sabatini DM (2009) mTOR signaling at a glance. *Journal of Cell Science* **122**(Pt 20): 3589–3594. doi: 10.1242/jcs.051011.

Larson K (2012) *Where the Heart Beats: John Cage, Zen Buddhism, and the Inner Life of Artists.* London: Penguin Books.

Lemon RN, Griffiths J (2005) Comparing the function of the corticospinal system in different species: organizational differences for motor specialization? *Muscle and Nerve* **32**(3): 261–279. doi: 10.1002/mus.20333.

Lexell J, Sjostrom M, Nordlund A-S, Taylor CC (1992) Growth and development of human muscle: a quantitative morphological study of whole vastus lateralis from childhood to adult age. *Muscle & Nerve* **15**(3): 404–409. doi: 10.1002/mus.880150323.

Liepert J, Tegenthoff M, Malin JP (1995) Changes of cortical motor area size during immobilization. *Electroencephalography and Clinical Neurophysiology* **97**(6): 382–386. doi: 10.1016/0924-980x(95)00194-p.

Lindsey PA, Newhouse JP (1989) *Second Surgical Opinion Programs: A Review of the Literature*. Santa Monica, CA: Rand Corp.

Lloyd S, Pagels H (1988) Complexity as thermodynamic depth. *Annals of Physics* **188**(1): 186–213.

Loewenstein WR (1999) *The Touchstone of Life: Molecular Information, Cell Communication, and the Foundations of Life*. Oxford: Oxford University Press.

Long YC, Glund S, Garcia-Roves PM, Zierath JR (2007) Calcineurin regulates skeletal muscle metabolism via coordinated changes in gene expression. *The Journal of Biological Chemistry* **282**(3): 1607–1614. doi: 10.1074/jbc.M609208200.

Lönnqvist P (2017) The potential implications of using disability-free survival and number needed to suffer as outcome measures for neonatal intensive care. *Acta Paediatrica* **107**(2): 200–202.

Lorentzen J, Willerslev-Olsen M, Hüche Larsen H, Farmer SF, Nielsen JB (2019) Maturation of feedforward toe walking motor program is impaired in children with cerebral palsy. *Brain: A Journal of Neurology* **142**(3): 526–541. doi: 10.1093/brain/awz002.

Macdonald H, Kontulainen S, Petit M, Janssen P, McKay H (2006) Bone strength and its determinants in pre- and early pubertal boys and girls. *Bone* **39**(3): 598–608. doi: 10.1016/j.bone.2006.02.057.

Malhotra S, Pandyan AD, Day CR, Jones PW, Hermens H (2009) Spasticity, an impairment that is poorly defined and poorly measured. *Clinical Rehabilitation* **23**(7): 651–658. doi: 10.1177/0269215508101747.

Mammucari C, Gherardi G, Zamparo I et al. (2015) The mitochondrial calcium uniporter controls skeletal muscle trophism in vivo. *Cell Reports* **10**(8): 1269–1279. doi: 10.1016/j.celrep.2015.01.056.

Marshall G, Blacklock JWS, Cameron C et al. (1948) Streptomycin treatment of pulmonary tuberculosis. *British Medical Journal* **2**(4582): 769 LP–782. doi: 10.1136/bmj.2.4582.769.

Martin E (2009) The Greeks may have had the last word, but who has the first? *Historia Medicinae* **1**(2). Available at: https://sites.google.com/a/medicinae.org/historia-medicinae/e111 (Accessed: 26 July 2021).

Martin JH (2005a) The corticospinal system: from development to motor control. *The Neuroscientist: A Review Journal Bringing Neurobiology, Neurology and Psychiatry* **11**(2): 161–173. doi: 10.1177/1073858404270843.

Martin JH (2005b) The corticospinal system: from development to motor control. *The Neuroscientist* **11**(2): 161–173.

Martin JH, Engber D, Meng Z (2005) Effect of forelimb use on postnatal development of the forelimb motor representation in primary motor cortex of the cat. *Journal of Neurophysiology* **93**(5): 2822–2831. doi: 10.1152/jn.01060.2004.

McCormack S, McCarthy M, Farilla L et al. (2011) Skeletal muscle mitochondrial function is associated with longitudinal growth velocity in children and adolescents. *The Journal of Clinical Endocrinology and Metabolism* **96**(10): E1612-8. doi: 10.1210/jc.2011-1218.

McCormick R, Vasilaki A (2018) Age-related changes in skeletal muscle: changes to life-style as a therapy. *Biogerontology* **19**(6): 519–536. doi: 10.1007/s10522-018-9775-3.

McLaughlin J (2017) The medical reshaping of disabled bodies as a response to stigma and a route to normality. *Medical Humanities* **43**(4): 244–250. doi: 10.1136/medhum-2016-011065.

Menconi MJ, Arany ZP, Alamdari N et al. (2010) Sepsis and glucocorticoids downregulate the expression of the nuclear cofactor PGC-1beta in skeletal muscle. *American Journal of Physiology. Endocrinology and Metabolism* **299**(4): E533–543. doi: 10.1152/ajpendo.00596.2009.

Merleau-Ponty M (1968) *The Visible and the Invisible*. Evanston, IL: Northwestern University Press.

Merleau-Ponty M (1988) *In Praise of Philosophy and Other Essays*. Evanston, IL: Northwestern University Press.

Merleau-Ponty M (2002) *The Phenomenology of Perception*. London: Routledge & Kegan Paul.

Milne N (2016) Curved bones: an adaptation to habitual loading. *Journal of Theoretical Biology* **407**: 18–24. doi: 10.1016/j.jtbi.2016.07.019.

Modlesky CM, Kanoff SA, Johnson DL, Subramanian P, Miller F (2009) Evaluation of the femoral midshaft in children with cerebral palsy using magnetic resonance imaging. *Osteoporos Int* **20**: 609–615.

Moore MJ, Rebeiz JJ, Holden M, Adams RD (1971) Biometric analyses of normal skeletal muscle. *Acta Neuropathologica* **19**(1): 51–69. doi: 10.1007/BF00690954.

Moran D (2011) Revisiting Sartre's ontology of embodiment in being and nothingness. In: Petrov V, editor, *Ontological Landscapes: Recent Thought on Conceptual Interfaces between Science and Philosophy*. Frankfurt: Ontos Verlag, pp. 263–294.

Morgan JD, Somerville EW (1960) Normal and abnormal growth at the upper end of the femur. *The Journal of Bone and Joint Surgery* **42-B**: 264–272. doi: 10.1302/0301-620X.42B2.264.

Mukund K, Mathewson M, Minamoto V, Ward SR, Subramaniam S, Lieber RL (2014) Systems analysis of transcriptional data provides insights into muscle's biological response to botulinum toxin. *Muscle & Nerve* **50**(5): 744–758. doi: 10.1002/mus.24211.

Mulderij KJ (2000) Dualistic notions about children with motor disabilities: hands to lean on or to reach out? *Qualitative Health Research* **10**(1): 39–50. doi: 10.1177/104973200129118237.

Navarrete R, Vrbová G (1993) Activity-dependent interactions between motoneurones and muscles: their role in the development of the motor unit. *Progress in Neurobiology* **41**(1): 93–124. doi: 10.1016/0301-0082(93)90041-p.

Neisser U (1988) Five kinds of self-knowledge. *Philosophical Psychology* **1**(1): 35–59.

Nicholson S, Kim E (2016) Structures in sound: analysis of classical music using the information length. *Entropy* **18**(7): 258.

Niescier RF, Kwak SK, Joo SH, Chang KT, Min KT (2016) Dynamics of mitochondrial transport in axons. *Frontiers in Cellular Neuroscience* **10**: 123. doi: 10.3389/fncel.2016.00123.

Nikolaou S, Peterson E, Kim A, Wylie C, Cornwall R (2011) Impaired growth of denervated muscle contributes to contracture formation following neonatal brachial plexus injury. *The Journal of Bone and Joint Surgery* **93**(5): 461–470. doi: 10.2106/JBJS.J.00943.

Nishimura T, Oyama K, Kishioka Y, Wakamatsu J, Hattori A (2007) Spatiotemporal expression of decorin and myostatin during rat skeletal muscle development. *Biochemical and Biophysical Research Communications* **361**(4): 896–902. doi: 10.1016/j.bbrc.2007.07.104.

Noble D (2012) A theory of biological relativity: no privileged level of causation. *Interface Focus* **2**(1): 55–64. doi: 10.1098/rsfs.2011.0067.

Noble JJ, Charles-Edwards DG, Keevil SF, Lewis AP, Gough M, Shortland AP (2014) Intramuscular fat in ambulant young adults with bilateral spastic cerebral palsy. *BMC Musculoskeletal Disorders* **15**(1): 1–8.

Noble JJ, Fry NR, Lewis AP et al. (2017) The relationship between lower limb muscle volume and body mass in ambulant individuals with bilateral cerebral palsy. *BMC Neurology* **17**(1): 1–9.

Nørretranders T (1991) *The User Illusion: Cutting Consciousness Down to Size*. New York: Viking.

Novak I, McIntyre S, Morgan C et al. (2013) A systematic review of interventions for children with cerebral palsy: state of the evidence. *Developmental Medicine and Child Neurology* **55**(10): 885–910. doi: 10.1111/dmcn.12246.

Nurse P (2008) Life, logic and information. *Nature* **454**(7203): 424–426.

Nussbaum MC (1986) *The Fragility of Goodness: Luck and Ethics in Greek Tragedy and Philosophy.* Cambridge: Cambridge University Press.

O'Sullivan MC, Eyre JA, Miller S (1991) Radiation of phasic stretch reflex in biceps brachii to muscles of the arm in man and its restriction during development. *The Journal of Physiology* **439**: 529–543. doi: 10.1113/jphysiol.1991.sp018680.

Oeffinger D, Bagley A, Rogers S et al. (2008) Outcome tools used for ambulatory children with cerebral palsy: responsiveness and minimum clinically important differences. *Developmental Medicine and Child Neurology* **50**(12): 918–925. doi: 10.1111/j.1469-8749.2008.03150.x.

Oertel G (1988) Morphometric analysis of normal skeletal muscles in infancy, childhood and adolescence. An autopsy study. *Journal of the Neurological Sciences* **88**(1–3): 303–313. doi: 10.1016/0022-510x(88)90227-4.

Osborne D, Effmann E, Broda K, Harrelson J (1980) The development of the upper end of the femur, with special reference to its internal architecture. *Radiology* **137**(1 Pt 1): 71–76. doi: 10.1148/radiology.137.1.7422864.

Otto A, Patel K (2010) Signalling and the control of skeletal muscle size. *Experimental Cell Research* **316**(18): 3059–3066. doi: 10.1016/j.yexcr.2010.04.009.

Pandyan A, Gregoric M, Barnes M et al. (2005) Spasticity: clinical perceptions, neurological realities and meaningful measurement. *Disability and Rehabilitation* **27**(1–2): 2–6. doi: 10.1080/09638280400014576.

Parkkinen VP, Wallmann C, Wilde M et al. (2018) *Evaluating Evidence of Mechanisms in Medicine: Principles and Procedures.* Cham: Springer Nature.

Pearl J (2010) An introduction to causal inference. *The International Journal of Biostatistics* **6**(2): Article 7. Available at: http://www.pubmedcentral.nih.gov/articlerender.fcgi?artid=2836213&tool= pmcentrez&rendertype=abstract.

Pette D, Staron RS (2000) Myosin isoforms, muscle fiber types, and transitions. *Microscopy Research and Technique* **50**(6): 500–509. doi: 10.1002/1097-0029(20000915)50:6<500::AID-JEMT7>3.0. CO;2-7.

Pingel J, Nielsen MS, Lauridsen T et al. (2017) Injection of high dose botulinum-toxin A leads to impaired skeletal muscle function and damage of the fibrilar and non-fibrilar structures. *Scientific Reports* **7**(1): 14746. doi: 10.1038/s41598-017-14997-3.

Polanyi M (1962) *Personal Knowledge: Towards a Post-critical Philosophy* (rev. ed.). London: Routledge & Kegan Paul.

Popper K (2002) *The Logic of Scientific Discovery.* London: Routledge.

Prechtl HFR (1993) Principles of early motor development in the human. In: Kalverboer AF, Hopkins B, Gueze R, editors, *Motor Development in Early and Later Childhood: Longitudinal Approaches.* Cambridge: Cambridge University Press, pp. 35–50.

Purslow PP (2002) The structure and functional significance of variations in the connective tissue within muscle. *Comparative Biochemistry and Physiology. Part A Molecular & Integrative Physiology* **133**(4): 947–966. doi: 10.1016/s1095-6433(02)00141-1.

Rauch F (2005) Bone growth in length and width: the yin and yang of bone stability. *Journal of Musculoskeletal & Neuronal Interactions* **5**(3): 194–201.

Reedman SE, Boyd RN, Elliott C, Sakzewski L (2017) ParticiPAte CP: a protocol of a randomised waitlist controlled trial of a motivational and behaviour change therapy intervention to increase physical activity through meaningful participation in children with cerebral palsy. *BMJ Open* **7**(8): e015918. doi: 10.1136/bmjopen-2017-015918.

Richards DW (1961) The first aphorism of Hippocrates. *Perspectives in Biology and Medicine* **5**: 61–64. doi: 10.1353/pbm.1961.0020.

Richter EA, Mikines KJ, Galbo H, Kiens B (1989) Effect of exercise on insulin action in human skeletal muscle. *Journal of Applied Physiology* **66**(2): 876–885.

Rochat P (2011) What is it like to be a newborn? In: Gallagher S, editor, *The Oxford Handbook of the Self*. Oxford: Oxford University Press, pp. 57–79.

Rosenbaum P, Gorter JW (2012) The 'F-words' in childhood disability: I swear this is how we should think! *Child: Care, Health and Development* **38**(4): 457–463. doi: 10.1111/j.1365-2214.2011.01338.x.

Runge J, Bathiany S, Bollt E et al. (2019) Inferring causation from time series in Earth system sciences. *Nat Commun* **10**: 2553. https://doi.org/10.1038/s41467-019-10105-3.

Russo F, Williamson J (2007) Interpreting causality in the health sciences. *International Studies in the Philosophy of Science* **21**(2): 157–170. doi: 10.1080/02698590701498084.

Rutkow IM, Gittelsohn AM, Zuidema GD (1979) Surgical decision making. The reliability of clinical judgment. *Annals of Surgery* **190**(3): 409–419. doi: 10.1097/00000658-197909000-00017.

Sackett DL, Rosenberg WMC, Gray JAM, Haynes RB, Richardson WS. (1996) Evidence based medicine: what it is and what it isn't. *BMJ (Clinical Research Ed.)* **312**(7023): 71–72. doi: 10.1136/bmj.312.7023.71.

Sapir E (1929) The status of linguistics as a science. *Language*. JSTOR: 207–214.

Sartre, J-P (1983) *Being and Nothingness: A Phenomenological Essay on Ontology*. Translator Hazel Barnes, New York: Pocket.

Sartre J-P (1989) Existentialism is a humanism. In: Kaufman W, editor, *Existentialism from Dostoyevsky to Sartre*. London: Meridian Publishing Company.

Saxton WM, Hollenbeck PJ (2012) The axonal transport of mitochondria. *Journal of Cell Science* **125**(Pt 9): 2095–2104. doi: 10.1242/jcs.053850.

Schiaffino S, Sandri M, Murgia M (2007) Activity-dependent signaling pathways controlling muscle diversity and plasticity. *Physiology* **22**: 269–278. doi: 10.1152/physiol.00009.2007.

Schiavio A, Maes P-J, van der Schyff D (2021) The dynamics of musical participation. *Musicae Scientiae*. London: Sage UK: England, p. 1029864920988319.

Schienda J, Engleka KA, Jun S et al. (2006) Somitic origin of limb muscle satellite and side population cells. *Proceedings of the National Academy of Sciences of the United States of America* **103**(4): 945–950. doi: 10.1073/pnas.0510164103.

Schloon H, Schlottmann J, Lenard HG, Goebel HH (1979) The development of skeletal muscles in premature infants. I. Fibre size and histochemical differentiation. *European Journal of Pediatrics* **131**(1): 49–60. doi: 10.1007/BF00442785.

Schmidt I, Herpin P (1997) Postnatal changes in mitochondrial protein mass and respiration in skeletal muscle from the newborn pig. *Comparative Biochemistry and Physiology. Part B, Biochemistry & Molecular Biology* **118**(3): 639–647. doi: 10.1016/s0305-0491(97)00268-x.

Scholtes VA, Becher JG, Beelen A, Lankhorst GJ (2006) Clinical assessment of spasticity in children with cerebral palsy: a critical review of available instruments. *Developmental Medicine and Child Neurology* **48**(1): 64–73. doi: 10.1017/S0012162206000132.

Schulz KF, Chalmers I, Hayes RJ, Altman DG (1995) Empirical evidence of bias: dimensions of methodological quality associated with estimates of treatment effects in controlled trials. *JAMA* **273**(5): 408–412. doi: 10.1001/jama.1995.03520290060030.

Schwartz MH, Rozumalski A, Truong W, Novacheck TF (2013) Predicting the outcome of intramuscular psoas lengthening in children with cerebral palsy using preoperative gait data and the random forest algorithm. *Gait & Posture* **37**(4): 473–479. doi: https://doi.org/10.1016/j.gaitpost.2012.08.016.

Serrano AL, Muñoz-Cánoves P (2010) Regulation and dysregulation of fibrosis in skeletal muscle. *Experimental Cell Research* **316**(18): 3050–3058. doi: 10.1016/j.yexcr.2010.05.035.

Shannon CE (1948) A mathematical theory of communication. *The Bell System Technical Journal* **27**(3): 379–423.

Shefelbine SJ, Carter DR (2004) Mechanobiological predictions of femoral anteversion in cerebral palsy. *Annals of Biomedical Engineering* **32**(2): 297–305. doi: 10.1023/b:abme.0000012750.73170.ba.

Shortland A (2009) Muscle deficits in cerebral palsy and early loss of mobility: can we learn something from our elders? *Developmental Medicine and Child Neurology* **51**: 59–63.

Simms E (1993) The infant's experience of the world: Stern, Merleau-Ponty and the phenomenology of the preverbal self. *The Humanistic Psychologist* **21**(1): 26–40.

Skaggs D, Rethlefsen SA, Kay RM, Dennis SW, Reynolds RAK, Tolo VT (2000) Variability in gait analysis interpretation. *Journal of Pediatric Orthopedics* **20**(6): 759–764. doi: 10.1097/00004694-200011000-00012.

Smil V (2017) *Energy: A Beginner's Guide.* New York: Simon and Schuster.

Smith LR, Pontén E, Hedström Y et al. (2009) Novel transcriptional profile in wrist muscles from cerebral palsy patients. *BMC Medical Genomics* **2**(1): 1–16.

Smith LR, Lee KS, Ward SR, Chambers HG, Lieber RL (2011) Hamstring contractures in children with spastic cerebral palsy result from a stiffer extracellular matrix and increased in vivo sarcomere length. *The Journal of Physiology* **589**(Pt 10): 2625–2639. doi: 10.1113/jphysiol.2010.203364.

Smith LR, Chambers HG, Subramaniam S et al. (2012) Transcriptional abnormalities of hamstring muscle contractures in children with cerebral palsy. *PloS One* **7**(8): e40686. doi: 10.1371/journal.pone.0040686.

Soo B, Howard JJ, Boyd RN et al. (2006) Hip displacement in cerebral palsy. *The Journal of Bone and Joint Surgery* **88**(1): 121–129. doi: 10.2106/JBJS.E.00071.

Specker BL, Schoenau E (2005) Quantitative bone analysis in children: current methods and recommendations. *Journal of Pediatrics* **146**(6): 726–731. doi: 10.1016/j.jpeds.2005.02.002.

Stackhouse SK, Binder-Macleod SA, Lee SCK (2005) Voluntary muscle activation, contractile properties, and fatigability in children with and without cerebral palsy. *Muscle and Nerve* **31**(5): 594–601. doi: 10.1002/mus.20302.

Stern DN (1990) *Diary of a Baby: What Your Child Sees, Feels, and Experiences.* New York: Basic Books.

Stevens TJ, Lando D, Basu S et al. (2017) 3D structures of individual mammalian genomes studied by single-cell Hi-C. *Nature* **544**(7648): 59–64. doi: 10.1038/nature21429.

Strauss D, Ojdana K, Shavelle R et al. (2004) Decline in function and life expectancy of older persons with cerebral palsy. *NeuroRehabilitation* **19**(1): 69–78. doi: 10.3233/nre-2004-19108.

Stuart CA, Shangraw RE, Prince MJ, Wolfe RR (1988) Bed-rest-induced insulin resistance occurs primarily in muscle. *Metabolism* **37**(8): 802–806.

Suryawan A, Orellana RA, Nguyen HV, Jeyapalan AS, Fleming JR, Davis TA (2007) Activation by insulin and amino acids of signaling components leading to translation initiation in skeletal muscle of neonatal pigs is developmentally regulated. *American Journal of Physiology. Endocrinology and Metabolism* **293**(6): E1597-605. doi: 10.1152/ajpendo.00307.2007.

Sutherland D, Olshen R, Biden E, Wyatt MP (1988) *The Development of Mature Walking.* Cambridge: Cambridge University Press.

Tarnas R (1996) *The Passion of the Western Mind: Understanding the Ideas That Have Shaped Our World View.* London: Pimlico.

Tedroff K, Granath F, Forssberg H, Haglund-Akerlind Y (2009) Long-term effects of botulinum toxin A in children with cerebral palsy. *Developmental Medicine and Child Neurology* **51**(2): 120–127. doi: 10.1111/j.1469-8749.2008.03189.x.

Tedroff K, Hägglund G, Miller F (2020) Long-term effects of selective dorsal rhizotomy in children with cerebral palsy: a systematic review. *Developmental Medicine and Child Neurology* **62**(5): 554–562. doi: 10.1111/dmcn.14320.

Thorn SR, Regnault TRH, Brown LD et al. (2009) Intrauterine growth restriction increases fetal hepatic gluconeogenic capacity and reduces messenger ribonucleic acid translation initiation and nutrient sensing in fetal liver and skeletal muscle. *Endocrinology* **150**(7): 3021–3030. doi: 10.1210/en.2008-1789.

Towers HM, Schulze KF, Ramakrishnan R, Kashyap S (1997) Energy expended by low birth weight infants in the deposition of protein and fat. *Pediatric Research* **41**(4 Pt 1): 584–589. doi: 10.1203/00006450-199704000-00021.

Ulrich W (2005) A brief introduction to critical systems heuristics (CSH). *ECOSENSUS project website,* The Open University, Milton Keynes, UK, 14 October 2005. http://projects.kmi.open.ac.uk/ecosensus/publications/ulrich_csh_intro.pdf.

Ulrich W, Reynolds M (2010) Critical systems heuristics. In: Reynolds M, Holwell S, editors, *Systems Approaches to Managing Change: A Practical Guide*. London: Springer, pp. 243–292.

Urso ML, Scrimgeour AG, Chen YW, Thompson PD, Clarkson PM (2006) Analysis of human skeletal muscle after 48 h immobilization reveals alterations in mRNA and protein for extracellular matrix components. *Journal of Applied Physiology* **101**(4): 1136–1148. doi: 10.1152/japplphysiol.00180.2006.

Vinay L, Brocard F, Clarac F, Noreel JC, Pearlstein E, Pflieger JF (2002) Development of posture and locomotion: an interplay of endogenously generated activities and neurotrophic actions by descending pathways. *Brain Research Reviews* **40**(1–3): 118–129. doi: 10.1016/S0165-0173(02)00195-9.

von Walden F, Gantelius S, Liu C et al. (2018) Muscle contractures in patients with cerebral palsy and acquired brain injury are associated with extracellular matrix expansion, pro-inflammatory gene expression, and reduced rRNA synthesis. *Muscle & Nerve* **58**(2): 277–285. doi: 10.1002/mus.26130.

Wallace DC, Fan W (2010) Energetics, epigenetics, mitochondrial genetics. *Mitochondrion* **10**(1): 12–31. doi: 10.1016/j.mito.2009.09.006.

Wang Z (2018) Antisense RNA and cancer. In: Chakrabarti J, Mitra S, editors, *Translational Epigenetics, Cancer and Noncoding RNAs*. Cambridge, MA: Academic Press, pp. 203–227.

Webber CE, Barr RD (2012) Age- and gender-dependent values of skeletal muscle mass in healthy children and adolescents. *Journal of Cachexia, Sarcopenia and Muscle* **3**(1): 25–29. doi: 10.1007/s13539-011-0042-6.

Welsh T (2013) *The Child as Natural Phenomenologist: Primal and Primary Experience in Merleau-Ponty's Psychology*. Evanston, IL: Northwestern University Press.

Westerblad H, Bruton JD, Katz A (2010) Skeletal muscle: energy metabolism, fiber types, fatigue and adaptability. *Experimental Cell Research* **316**(18): 3093–3099. doi: 10.1016/j.yexcr.2010.05.019.

Wickiewicz TL, Roy RR, Powell PL, Edgerton VR (1983) Muscle architecture of the human lower limb. *Clinical Orthopaedics and Related Research* (179): 275–283.

Willerslev-Olsen M, Lorentzen J, Sinkjaer T, Nielsen JB (2013) Passive muscle properties are altered in children with cerebral palsy before the age of 3 years and are difficult to distinguish clinically from spasticity. *Developmental Medicine and Child Neurology* **55**(7): 617–623. doi: 10.1111/dmcn.12124.

Willerslev-Olsen M, Lund MC, Lorentzen J, Barber L, Kofoed-Hansen M, Nielson JB (2018) Impaired muscle growth precedes development of increased stiffness of the triceps surae musculotendinous unit in children with cerebral palsy. *Developmental Medicine and Child Neurology* **60**(7): 672–679. doi: 10.1111/dmcn.13729.

Williams TC, Bach CC, Matthiesen NB, Henriksen TB, Gagliardi L (2018) Directed acyclic graphs: a tool for causal studies in paediatrics. *Pediatric Research* **84**(4): 487–493. doi: 10.1038/s41390-018-0071-3.

Wilt TJ, Fink HA (2007) Systematic reviews and meta-analyses. *Clinical Research Methods for Surgeons* (February): 311–325. doi: 10.1007/978-1-59745-230-4_18.

Wingert JR, Sinclair RJ, Dixit S, Damiano DL, Burton H (2010) Somatosensory-evoked cortical activity in spastic diplegic cerebral palsy. *Human Brain Mapping* **31**(11): 1772–1785. doi: 10.1002/hbm.20977.

Wittgenstein L (1953) *Philosophical Investigations.* Oxford: Basil Blackwell.

Wittgenstein L (1969) *On Certainty.* Oxford: Basil Blackwell.

Wolpert DM, Diedrichsen J, Flanagan JR (2011) Principles of sensorimotor learning. *Nature Reviews. Neuroscience* **12**(12): 739–751. doi: 10.1038/nrn3112.

Wren TAL, Rethlefsen S, Kay RM (2005) Prevalence of specific gait abnormalities in children with cerebral palsy. *Journal of Pediatric Orthopaedics* **25**(1): 79–83. doi: 10.1097/01241398-200501000-00018.

Wright S (1932) *The Role of Mutation, Inbreeding, Crossbreeding and Selection in Evolution.* Sixth International Congress of Genetics. Brooklyn, NY: Brooklyn Botanical Garden.

Yao, KT, Chang M-H (1993) Growth and body composition of preterm, small-for-gestational age infants at a postmenstrual age of 37–40 weeks. *Early Hum Dev* **33**: 117–131.

Zhu J, Li Y, Shen W et al. (2007) Relationships between transforming growth factor-beta1, myostatin, and decorin: implications for skeletal muscle fibrosis. *The Journal of Biological Chemistry* **282**(35): 25852–25863. doi: 10.1074/jbc.M704146200.

Index

A

acetylcholine binds, 67
acetyl-CoA acetylates, 62
acetyl-Coenzyme A (acetyl-CoA), 59
    citrate, 59
    four-carbon molecule, 59
adenosine diphosphate (ADP), 59
adenosine monophosphate (AMP), 59
adenosine triphosphate (ATP), 55, 134
    citrate lyase, 62
    formation of, 60
    synthase, 60, 61
algorithmic information content (AIC), 82, 83, 130
alpha motor neuron (αMN), 72, 75
AMP-activated protein kinase (AMPK), 63, 77, 97
ascertainment bias, 37
Assisting Hand Assessment (AHA), 107, 108
axon, 73–77, 88–90

B

Bach, Johann Sebastian, 49
Bayesian methods, 34
Being and Nothingness (Sartre), 142
belief, disconfirmation of, 17–18
Berger's concept, of the nomos, 20
bias
    anchoring, 8
    availability, 8
    commission, 8
    confirmation, 8
    Festinger's conditions, 18
    randomised controlled trial, 37–39
    representativeness, 8
bilateral cerebral palsy, 2
    5-year-old boy
        hip development, 2, 151
        hip dysplasia, 2

    12-year-old boy, 3, 152
    physiotherapist, 150
bone, remodelling of, 64
botulinum toxin
    botulinum toxin (BTX), 122
    botulinum toxin A (BTX-A), 106
    muscle denervation, 18
brain glucose demand, 87

C

calcium, mitochondrial uptake of, 71
Canadian Occupational Performance Measure (COPM), 28, 39, 106
cancellous bone, remodelling of, 64
Carroll, Lewis, 15
causal loop diagrams, 85–87, 90, 93, 100, 136, 154
cell cytoskeleton, 63
cell development, epigenetics/state space/ adaptive possible, 79–80
cell membrane, 57
cell metabolism, 61
cells expression, 63
cellular proteins, 57
cerebral palsy, 114
    in 8-year-old boy, 2
    in 4-year-old girl, 2
    bilateral cerebral palsy, 2
    care of children, 13, 147
    clinical model of, 1
    complication, 152–153
    consistency, lack of, 15
    failure of belief, 17–18
    management, by medical student, 12
    muscular strength/control, 116
    musculoskeletal deformity, in children, 16
    musculoskeletal development, in children, 95–96
    musculoskeletal system, clinical management of, 11

philosophical analysis of, 5
physiotherapist, 1, 2, 149
randomised controlled trials
    acknowledging, 114–117
    analogy, 114
    application of, 106–109
    association strength, 111–112
    biological gradient/dose-response
        relationship, 112–113
    coherence, 113
    consistency, 112
    experiment, 113
    hypotheses and outcome measures,
        109–110
    plausibility, 113
    problem solving, 104–117
    research studies, lack of, 111–114
    specificity, 112
    temporality, 112
    treatments, evaluation of, 110–111
role of paradigm, 19–21
skeletal muscle function, 148
treatments, evidence base, 123–124
children
    development, 135
    musculoskeletal management, 21, 24
    quality of life, 26
chronic spinal cord injury, 71
Clausius, Rudolph, 51
clinical decision-making, 21, 22, 124, 132, 136,
    137, 141, 146, 152
clinical knowledge, 126
    concept of, 126–127
    Cynefin framework, 127–131
    systems approach, 133–135
    uncertainty, 131–133
clinically significant improvement, 36–37
Cochrane Methodology Review Group, 118
codified knowledge, 10–11, 13, 20–21, 24
codons, in DNA code, 58
coenzyme A (CoA), 59
cognitive characteristics, 29
cognitive dissonance, role of, 17–18
cognitive ease, 8, 17
cognitive strain, 8
constraint-induced movement therapy
    (CIMT), 107
corps objectif, 26, 142
cortical bone, 64

corticospinal tract, role of, 89–90
critical systems heuristics (CSH), 137–141
Cynefin framework, 127–129
    clinical knowledge and, 130–131

D

Delphi method, 35
dendrites, 73–74
denkkolectiv, 19
denkstil, 19
deoxyribonucleic acid (DNA), 58
    codons, 58
    methylation, 62, 96
    transcription, 62
Derrida, Jacques, 19
directed acyclic graphs (DAGs), 118, 119
    collider, 121
    confounders, 118–120
    mediators, 120–121
    using/validating, 121–123
dose-response curve, 113
drug's side-effects, 38
Duheim-Quine thesis/problem, 18
dynamical depth, 53–54, 82, 130

E

Einstein's theory of relativity, 20
electrical stimulation, 71, 120, 123
energy flow, in cells, 60–61
entropy, 52
    developmental trajectories, 83–84
    Shannon concept of, 53
enzymes, 57
epistemology, 6
eukaryotic cell, 57
evidence-based knowledge, 12
evidence-based medicine (EBM), 104, 123
    cerebral palsy, 102, 103
    childhood cancer/asthma, treatment of,
        102
    clinical experience, 103–104
    definition of, 10
    observational studies, 117–118
    weaknesses of, 117
excitatory postsynaptic potentials (EPSPs), 73

F

fibroadipogenic progenitors (FAPs), 97
fibrosis, 97
Fleck, Ludwik, 19
follow-up, short-term, 39–40
Food and Drug Administration (FDA), 30
free energy, 60

G

gastro-oesophageal reflux, 3
gene expression, in muscles of children, 95
gene regulatory network, 80
glycolysis, 59, 70
God of Earth, 17
Golgi apparatus, 60
Golgi tendon organ, 75
Grading of Recommendations, Assessment,
    Development, and Evaluations (GRADE)
    system, 105
Gross Motor Function Classification System
    (GMFCS), 139
Gross Motor Function Measure (GMFM), 31,
    36, 39, 42
Gross Motor Function Measure-66
    (GMFM-66), 28, 29

H

hip dysplasia
    5-year-old boy, 2
    in children, 98
    management of, 3
hip joint development, 94
human musculoskeletal system.
    See musculoskeletal system
Husserl, Edmund, 25
hydroxyapatite ($Ca_{10}(PO_4)_6(OH)_2$), 64
Hypothesising After the Results are Known
    (HARKing), 109

I

inhibitory postsynaptic potentials (IPSPs), 73
International Classification of Functioning,
    Disability and Health (ICF), 126
intrafusal fibres, 75

J

junk DNA, 58

K

Kant, Immanuel, 6
knee joint, in humans, 69
knowledge
    clinical, 126–127 (*See also* Clinical
        knowledge)
    codified, 10
    Cynefin framework, 127–130
    defined, 9–11
    evidence-based, 12
    lack of, 24
    pretheoretical, 13
    tacit, 10, 13
    transfer, 106
    types of, 9
Krebs cycle, 60
Kuhn, Thomas, 19–21

L

language game, 14
language habits, 11
leptin, 77
lifespan model, 117
limb alignment, 100–101
limb immobilisation, 71
lived-in body, 26–27
    child's objective body, 26
    musculoskeletal system, 145–146
living systems, 52
Logic of Scientific Discovery, The, 10

M

magnetic resonance imaging (MRI), 93
mechanistic target of rapamycin (mTOR),
    62
Medical Research Council, 30
messenger RNA (mRNA), 58
    codon sequence in DNA, 58
    ribosome binds, 58

minimal clinically important difference
    (MCID), 35, 36
minimal detectable difference (MDD), 44
mitogen-activated protein kinase, 62
Modified Ashworth Scale, 30
Modified Tardieu Scale (MTS) score, 29, 38, 43
motor control
    after birth, 90–91
    movement, 90–91
motor neurons, upper/lower, concept of, 75
motor unit (MU), 72
mTOR pathway, 77
muscle
    architecture, 68–69
    contraction begins, 89
    cross-sectional area (MCSA), 93
    denervation, 18, 71
    developmental pathways, 99
    function, 68–69
    growth, 16
    innervation, 72–73
    protein synthesis, 72, 92
    'slow'/'fast', 70
muscle fibre, 16, 71
    development, 92
    factors influencing, 92
    growth, 91–92
    hypertrophy, 95
    phenotype, 87
    'slow-twitch', 70
muscular strength/control, 115
musculectomy, 43
musculoskeletal deformity, 16, 21–23, 26, 81,
    102, 133, 146, 149–150
musculoskeletal development
    algorithmic information content (AIC),
        82, 83
    causal loop diagram, 85
    cerebral palsy, in children, 95–96
    changes, 96–99
    clinical practice, 136–137
    critical systems heuristics (CSH),
        137–141
    developmental trajectories, 81
    external factors, role of, 135–136
    interactive pathways, 91
    loop diagrams, 100–101
    potential trajectories, 81
    thermodynamical depth, 82

musculoskeletal system, 48, 50
    ATP, enzymatic breakdown of, 59
    causal loop diagrams, 85–87
    cell membrane, 56
    cellos/muscles, 48–49
    cellular energy balance, 61–62
    changes, 96–99
    children, with cerebral palsy, 99
    clinical knowledge, 146
    clinical management of, 141
    component systems, 51
    concept of, 101
    defined, 46–47
    development (See musculoskeletal
        development)
    difficulties, 84–85
    DNA, for transcription/gene expression, 63
    embryo development, 88–89
    energy costs, 87
    entropy/developmental trajectories, 83–84
    entropy/information/cell, 51–56
    framework, 63–65
    growth, 80–83
    interactive pathways, 94
    linear/nonlinear, 47
    lived-in body, 145–146
        clinical relevance of, 143–144
        Maurice Merleau-Ponty's concept of,
            142–143
    mitochondrion, cell's power station, 59–61
    and movement, 51
    muscle contraction
        begins early, 89
        components of, 66–67
        molecular basis, 67–68
    muscle developmental pathways, 99
    myocyte, 65–66
    orchestra playing music, 49–50
    prime mover, 65
    proteins, 56–59
    Sartre's view, 141–142
    severe cognitive impairment, 144–145
    skill/ability, 50
    systemic energy balance, 62–63
myelin, 74
myoblasts, 115
myocyte development, 65, 66, 86
myofibrils, 66, 113, 116
myosin heavy chain (MHC) isoform, 70

N

National Council for Clinical Advice (NCCA), 40–42
neonatal brachial plexus palsy, mouse models of, 92
neonatal skeletal muscle, 83
nerve cell membrane, 73, 74
nervous system
    central nervous system, 75–76
    movement control, 72
    neuron, 72–73
    neuronal signalling, basis of, 73–74
neuromuscular electrical stimulation, 71
neuronal signalling
    basis of, 73–74
    neuron, energy needs of, 74–75
Newtonian model of reality, 20
Nicomachean Ethics, 9, 132
nicotinamide adenine dinucleotide (NAD), 60

O

odds ratio (OR), 34, 35, 107
on-going therapy, 39
ontologic/aleatory uncertainty, 151
ontology, 6
osteocalcin, 77

P

paediatric neurodisability, 30
ParticiPAte trial, 111
perimysium, 66–67
p-hacking, 109–110
phosphatases, 57
phosphatidylinositol-3-kinase, 62
physiological cross-sectional area (PCSA), 69
physiotherapist, cerebral palsy, 1, 2, 149
plasticity, 84
Poisson distribution, 9
Polanyi, Michael, 10
postconception weeks (PCW) myoblasts, 88
pretheoretical knowledge, 13, 21, 25
proteins, 56
    cellular, 57
    muscle protein synthesis, 92
    synthesis, energy costs, 87

R

radiologist, 10
randomised controlled trial (RCT), 28, 30, 130
    advantage of, 119
    algorithm development, 34
    bias, 37–39
    cerebral palsy, problem solving, 104–117
    clinical guidelines, 40–44
    criterion standard, 30
    database studies, 34
    double-blinded, 37, 117
    internal validity, 32
    long-term outcomes, 39–40
    measuring outcomes, 42–44
    odds ratio (OR), 35
    outcome statistics, 30–37
    participants, 36
    physical activity (PA), 120
    RaSP-CP trial, 31–33
    relative risk, 34
    sample sizes, 30–37
    vulnerable to confounding, 119
RaSP-CP trial, 31–35, 37, 39
relative risk (RR), 34
ribonucleic acid (RNA) molecules, 58
Royal Society of Medicine, 111

S

sarcolemma, 65–67, 70, 73
sarcomere, contractile proteins of, 67
sensori-motor control, 14
sensory development, 98, 99
sensory information, structure, 6–8
shared decision-making model, 110–111
signalling pathways, within cell pass, 54
sirtuins, 62, 96
six-carbon sugars ($C_6H_{12}O_6$), 61
skeletal muscle
    balancing energy/growth, 77–78
    cell development, 90, 93–95
    dynamic/responsive, 70–72
    effect of, 93–95
    fibre growth/development, 91–92
    movement, concept of, 78
    part of, 76

social knowledge, 12
spasticity
    clinical method, 15
    concept of, 13–17
    definition of, 14, 15
    sensori-motor control, 14
Structure of Scientific Revolutions, The (1962), 19
surgical decision-making, 22

T

tacit knowledge, 10, 21, 25
Tardieu Scale, 29, 38, 43
T-cells system, 70
theoretical knowledge, 13, 25
Thompson, D'Arcy, 46
thought constraint, 19
Through the Looking-Glass, 15
tibialis anterior, denervation of, 71
troponin-C, on thin filament, 66, 68
T-tubules, 65–67

U

US Department of Health and Human Services
    on the Second Surgical Opinion Program, 22

V

voltage-gated ion channels, 67, 74

W

Waddington's model, epigenetic landscapes,
    80
Wittgenstein, Ludwig, 14
World Health Organization's International
    Classification of Functioning, Disability and
    Health (ICF), 43

X

X-ray absorptiometry, 98

Z

Zenetec, 28, 39
    injectable spasticity therapies, 40
    Joe's musculature, 44
    on muscle development, 40
    side-effects, 42

Other titles from Mac Keith Press

www.mackeith.co.uk

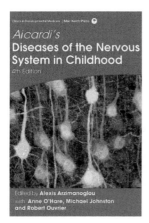

Aicardi's Diseases of the Nervous System in Childhood, 4th Edition

Alexis Arzimanoglou, Anne O'Hare, Michael V Johnston and Robert Ouvrier (Editors)

Clinics in Developmental Medicine
2018 ▪ 1524pp ▪ hardback ▪ 9781909962804

This fourth edition retains the patient-focussed, clinical approach of its predecessors. The international team of editors and contributors has honoured the request of the late Jean Aicardi, that his book remain 'resolutely clinical', which distinguishes *Diseases of the Nervous System in Childhood* from other texts in the field. New edition completely updated and revised and now in full colour.

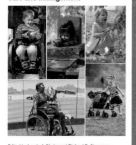

Children and Youth with Complex Cerebral Palsy: Care and Management

Laurie J Glader and Richard D Stevenson (Editors)

A Practical Guide from Mac Keith Press
2019 ▪ 404pp ▪ softback ▪ 9781909962989

This is the first practical guide to explore management of the many medical comorbidities that children with complex CP face, including orthopaedics, mobility needs, cognition and sensory impairment, difficult behaviours, respiratory complications and nutrition, amongst others. Uniquely, contributors include children and parents, providing applied wisdom for family-centred care. Clinical Care Tools are provided to help guide clinicians and include a Medical Review Supplement, Equipment and Services Checklist and an ICF-Based Care: Goals and Management Form.

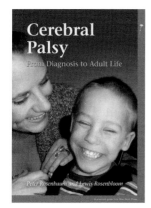

Cerebral Palsy: From Diagnosis to Adult Life

Peter L Rosenbaum, Lewis Rosenbloom (Authors)

A Practical Guide from Mac Keith Press
2012 ▪224pp ▪ softback ▪ 9781908316509

A highly readable and accessible overview of Cerebral Palsy. The book has been designed to provide readers with an understanding of Cerebral Palsy as a developmental as well as a neurological condition. It details the nature of Cerebral Palsy, its causes and its clinical manifestations. Using clear, accessible language (supported by an extensive glossary) the authors have blended current science with metaphor both to explain the biomedical underpinnings of Cerebral Palsy and to share their awareness that there is much that can be done to promote child and family development, enhance the capabilities of young people with Cerebral Palsy, empower their families, and chart a course into adulthood.

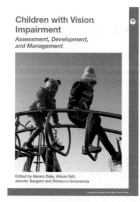

Children with Vision Impairment: Assessment, Development, and Management
Naomi Dale, Alison Salt, Jenefer Sargent, and Rebecca Greenaway (Editors)

Mac Keith Press Practical Guides
2021 ▪ 288pp ▪ softback▪ 9781911612339

Vision impairment is a long-term condition caused by disorders of the eye, optic nerve, and brain. Using evidence-based knowledge, theory, and research, this book provides practical guidance for practitioners who are involved in the care and management of children with long-term vision impairment and disability.

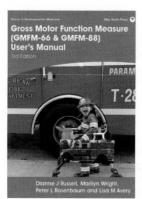

Gross Motor Function Measure (GMFM-66 & GMFM-88) User's Manual 3rd Edition
Dianne J Russell, Marilyn Wright, Peter L Rosenbaum, Lisa M Avery (Editors)

Clinics in Developmental Medicine
2021▪ 320pp ▪ softback ▪ 9781911612490

The third edition of the Gross Motor Function Measure (GMFM-66 & GMFM-88) User's Manual has retained the information contained in the original 2002 and 2013 publications which included the conceptual background to the development of the GMFM, and the administration and scoring guidelines for people to be able to administer this clinical and research assessment tool appropriately. The new edition contains updates and information on the GMFM App.

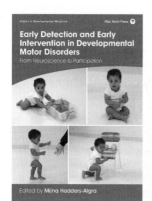

Early Detection and Early Intervention in Development Disorders: From Neuroscience to Participation
Mijna Hadders-Algra (Editor)

Clinics in Developmental Medicine
2021 ▪ 288pp ▪ hardback ▪ 9781911612438

The book provides a comprehensive overview of assessments and interventions applied in young children with or at high risk for developmental motor disorders. It provides an evidence-based practical guide for health professionals working in the field of early detection and early intervention.

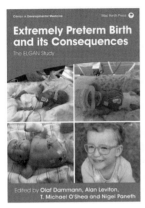

Extremely Preterm Birth and its Consequences: The ELGAN Study
Olaf Dammann, Alan Leviton, T Michael O'Shea, Nigel Paneth (Editors)

Clinics in Developmental Medicine
2020 ▪ 256pp ▪ hardback ▪ 9781911488965

The ELGAN (Extremely Low Gestational Age Newborns) Study was the largest and most comprehensive multicentre study ever completed for this population of babies born before 28 weeks' gestation. The authors' presentation and exploration of the results of the research will help clinicians to prevent adverse health outcomes and promote positive health for these children.

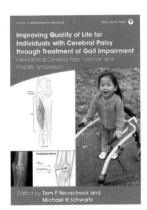

Improving Quality of Life for Individuals with Cerebral Palsy through Treatment of Gait Impairment
Tom Novacheck, Michael Schwartz (Editors)

Clinics in Developmental Medicine
2020 ▪ 163pp ▪ hardback ▪ 9781911612414

The *Symposium* brought together world-reknowned experts with a range of viewpoints to challenge each other and answer these questions, and prevent stagnation of outcomes. This publication unites these discussions to establish a framework to guide research efforts for the future and ensure meaningful progress. Authors consider how patient goals can be given more attention and ask how we can learn more details of the underlying neurological impairments.

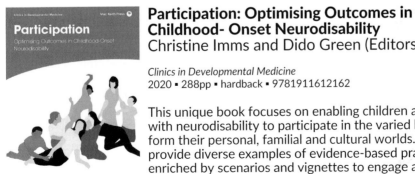

Participation: Optimising Outcomes in Childhood- Onset Neurodisability
Christine Imms and Dido Green (Editors)

Clinics in Developmental Medicine
2020 ▪ 288pp ▪ hardback ▪ 9781911612162

This unique book focuses on enabling children and young people with neurodisability to participate in the varied life situations that form their personal, familial and cultural worlds. Chapters provide diverse examples of evidence-based practices and are enriched by scenarios and vignettes to engage and challenge the reader to consider how participation in meaningful activities might be optimised for individuals and their families. The book's practical examples aim to facilitate knowledge transfer, clinical application and service planning for the future.

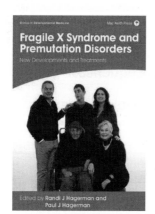

Fragile X Syndrome and Premutation Disorders: New Developments and Treatments
Randi J Hagerman, Paul J Hagerman (Editors)

Clinics in Developmental Medicine
2020 ▪ 192pp ▪ hardback▪ 9781911612377

Fragile X syndrome results from a gene mutation on the X-chromosome, which leads to various intellectual and developmental disabilities. Fragile X Syndrome and Premutation Disorders offers clinicians and families a multidisciplinary approach in order to provide the best possible care for patients with Fragile X. Unique features of the book include what to do when an infant or toddler is first diagnosed, the impact on the family and an international perspective on how different cultures perceive the syndrome.

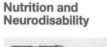
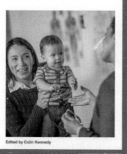

Nutrition and Neurodisability
Peter Sullivan, Guro Andersen, Morag Andrew (Editors)

Mac Keith Press Practical Guides
2020▪ 208pp ▪ softback ▪ 9781911612254

Feeding difficulties are common in children with neurodisability and disorders of the central nervous system can affect the movements required for safe and efficient eating and drinking. This practical guide provides strategies for managing the range of nutritional problems faced by children with neurodevelopmental disability.

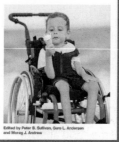

Principles and Practice of Child Neurology in Infancy, 2nd Edition
Colin Kennedy (Editor)

Mac Keith Press Practical Guides
2020 ▪ 552pp ▪ softback ▪ 9781911612001

Management of neurological disorders presenting in infancy poses many challenges for clinicians. Using a symptom-based approach, and covering a wide range of scenarios, the latest edition of this comprehensive practical guide provides authoritative advice from distinguished experts. It now includes revised coverage of disease prevention, clinical assessment, and promotion of neurodevelopment.